EATING WELL FOR A HEALTHY PREGNANCY

DR BARBARA PICKARD read Zoology at the University of Leeds and gained a PhD in reproductive physiology from the University of Nottingham. She is now a Honorary Research Fellow at the University of Leeds and is currently working on pregnancy sickness and pre-conception care. She lectures all over Britain to both professional and lay audiences, and has written numerous articles for magazines and journals, including *Mother* and *General Practitioner*. She has also broadcast on various television and radio programmes. Dr Pickard lives in Yorkshire, and is married with four children.

HEALTHCARE FOR WOMEN SERIES

Eating Well for a Healthy Pregnancy
Dr Barbara Pickard

Everything You Need to Know about the Pill
Wendy Cooper and Dr Tom Smith

Lifting the Curse
Beryl Kingston

Thrush
How it's caused and what to do about it
Caroline Clayton

Women and Depression
A practical self-help guide
Deidre Sanders

Women and Tranquillisers
Celia Haddon

Women's Problems: An A to Z
Dr Vernon Coleman

HEALTHCARE FOR WOMEN

EATING WELL FOR A HEALTHY PREGNANCY

Dr Barbara Pickard

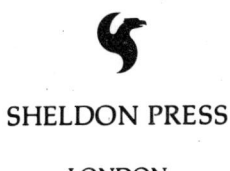

SHELDON PRESS

LONDON

First published in Great Britain in 1984 by
Sheldon Press, SPCK, Marylebone Road, London NW1 4DU

Copyright © Dr Barbara Pickard 1984

All rights reserved. No part of this book may be
reproduced or transmitted in any form or by any means,
electronic or mechanical, including photocopying,
recording, or by any information storage and retrieval
system, without permission in writing
from the publisher.

Note

Grams are used in the text for those foods commonly sold in
metric quantities, such as tinned and packaged food. Imperial
measurements (lbs and oz) are used for many foods bought
loose, such as meat and vegetables.

British Library Cataloguing in Publication Data

Pickard, Barbara
   Eating Well for a Healthy Pregnancy———(Healthcare
   for women)
   1. Pregnancy———Nutritional aspects
   I. Title   II. Series
   613.2'088042   RG559
ISBN 0-85969-416-X
ISBN 0-85969-417-8 Pbk

Photoset by Photobooks (Bristol) Ltd

Printed in Great Britain by
Richard Clay (The Chaucer Press) Ltd,
Bungay, Suffolk

Contents

1. It Takes Two   1
2. Healthy Eating   13
3. Does Weight Matter?   37
4. Putting Theory Into Practice   50
5. Nourishing Yourself and Your Baby   70
6. When It's Not So Easy   84
7. Special Needs   96
8. Happy Birthday – and Afterwards   108
9. Vitamins and Minerals   125
   Reading List   142
   List of Useful Addresses   147
   Index   151

ONE

It Takes Two

*'Peter and Anne are happy to
announce the arrival of baby John
on May 14th weighing 8 lb 1 oz'*

Having a baby is a very commonplace event – about three quarters of a million babies are born in the United Kingdom every year. Yet the birth of each and every child is still a very special occasion. Peter and Anne are happy because together they have created a new and unique individual. They are especially happy because they have a lovely, healthy baby. The majority of babies *are* normal, yet one of the first questions that Anne probably asked after the birth was 'Is the baby all right?' What is so remarkable about the immensely complex process which starts with sperm and egg and culminates in a newborn baby is that it goes to plan as often as it does.

How a baby develops

If the subject of baby development is entirely new to you, it may help to compare it to a very much simpler process, that of building a house. First essentials include a plan and some firm foundations. Only then can the raw materials, the stone, brick, wood, glass, pipes and wires be assembled and the workmen and their tools brought to the site. Also, there must be an effective communications system and facilities for the disposal of waste.

In the case of a baby, the egg and sperm jointly carry the 'plan' in special structures called the chromosomes. This plan will not only be influenced by the genetic backgrounds of both father and mother (which, in turn, were inherited from their own parents), but possibly also by their lifestyles. The 'foundations' for a baby's healthy development are the body and womb (uterus) of the prospective mother, and at monthly intervals the womb prepares itself in readiness for a possible embryo (a baby in the first few weeks of development).

When sperm and egg fuse together, the instructions in the plan are combined in a complex manner and the resulting information passed on to all the cells of the baby. Then the mother's body provides the major 'raw materials', the 'workmen' and their 'tools'.

Much of what you eat is made up of the major or 'macro' nutrients – the proteins, fats and carbohydrates – and these three groups of substances will supply most of the needs for building new tissues and for energy. The 'workmen' are special proteins called enzymes which help to construct the new tissues which will form the baby's body. Their 'tools' are the vitamins and minerals obtained from the foods you eat, and these will fulfil a wide variety of roles during the baby's development. Vitamin B_6, for example, among other functions, helps the worker enzymes to put together the protein components (amino acids) to build new tissue. Each slice of the wholemeal bread that you eat supplies a miniscule but meaningful amount of this vitamin. The cells of new tissues need to be held together with a kind of intercellular 'cement', and one of the many roles of vitamin C is to ensure that this cementing is done properly. When you eat an orange, the minute fraction which is vitamin C may be contributing to the integrity of your baby's tissues. Folate (sometimes called folic acid), a vitamin found in dark green vegetables, is needed for the healthy production of red blood cells and for the development of the nervous system.

When minerals are mentioned most people think of calcium and iron; calcium forms an essential part of bones and teeth and iron is a major constituent of haemoglobin, the substance in blood which will carry oxygen to the baby. However, these are but two minerals; there are others that have equally important functions (see Chapter 9).

The first twelve weeks
When the embryo is still only a few millimetres in size, your body begins to anticipate the demands which will be placed upon it in a few months time. Fat begins to be stored. This

It Takes Two

will be needed in late pregnancy when the baby's weight is increasing rapidly and also after the birth to help provide a good supply of milk. Your blood will have a lot of extra work to do during pregnancy – for example, transporting oxygen and nutrients, and removing waste products. Your circulatory system begins to make adjustments early in pregnancy. The total volume of blood and the number of red blood cells increase. Your endocrine or hormonal system adapts to the pregnant condition and new hormones, specific to pregnancy, are produced.

Your digestive system also alters during the early months. Your stomach becomes more sluggish and secretes less acid; the general movement of food through your intestines slows down. Some people think these changes allow for greater absorption of nutrients, others that they are merely the consequence of altered hormone levels. However, they sometimes have unfortunate side-effects: such as pregnancy sickness, heartburn or constipation. Your respiratory system and kidneys begin to work harder, in readiness for the need to supply more oxygen and to remove extra waste products. This can help to explain the need, by some mothers-to-be, for frequent visits to the toilet even in the early stages of pregnancy.

While all these changes are going on in your body, the baby is undergoing a crucial stage of development. The major parts of the body (the heart, brain, eyes, ears and other organs, the arms and legs, fingers and toes) are forming, so that by twelve weeks your baby has a well-defined human form, down to the last toenail.

Further growth

After this time, the major needs are for further growth and maturation. In order to cope with the great coming and going of substances to and from the developing baby, the placenta has evolved. This lifeline between you and the baby, formed during the first few months of pregnancy, is the means by which nutrients, oxygen and hormones are exchanged between you both, and waste products removed.

It hardly seems possible that your body could provide all the substances needed for building the new tissues of the baby and for constructing the placenta, making enzymes and hormones, supplying energy and oxygen and disposing of waste. Yet it can work in a beautifully coordinated manner right through pregnancy to ensure that everything goes according to plan, a plan requiring only the simplest of essentials from the environment around you – good food, water and oxygen.

The importance of sensible eating

Each item of food you eat is broken down by your digestive system into easily transportable substances, which are then absorbed into the bloodstream and used as needed or put into your body's 'stores' as a reserve supply of important nutrients. What these stores contain depends on how well you have been eating even before your baby was conceived. If some nutrients are in short supply from what you eat during pregnancy – during a period of morning sickness for instance, the baby can usually draw upon these emergency stores – provided they are adequate. Whatever the nutrient and whether it is required in large or small amounts, if it is seriously lacking things can go wrong. Your baby's development may be affected just a little or it may come to a complete halt.

If you are not interested in what you eat you may be sceptical about the need for a well-balanced diet in order to produce a healthy baby. Perhaps you feel well on a somewhat inadequate diet and think 'Why should my baby be any different?' But there *is* a difference between what adults need and what babies need. Adults need food for maintenance, not for growth and development. It can take years for the effect of an inadequate diet to show up in the health of an adult. If a grown-up eats poorly for a while and then eats well again, the damage can often be rectified and health returns to normal. In contrast, the period when a baby is developing is one when nutritional needs are great and it may not be possible for the effects of any inadequacy to be remedied. If a nutritional deficiency takes its toll at a critical stage of development, there is no turning the clock back.

It Takes Two

The evidence

Doubters may still say 'But what evidence is there that nutrition is so important, both before as well as during pregnancy?' Until relatively recently, most of this evidence came from work with animals. It has long been good husbandry practice among farmers and animal breeders to feed both male and female animals well and get them in good condition before mating, in addition to providing good food for the mother during pregnancy and lactation. Scientific experiments with animals have demonstrated the tragic effects of starving the mother or of feeding her a diet lacking in one or more important vitamins or minerals. She may fail to become pregnant at all. If she does conceive, she may be more likely to miscarry or some of the offspring may be born dead, deformed or too small.

Similar feeding experiments with human beings obviously could not take place. Nevertheless, history has provided us with situations almost like 'natural' experiments. For example, during the Nazi occupation of the Netherlands in World War II, there were severe famine conditions in some parts of the country. The Dutch Hunger Winter, as it was called, began in October 1944 and lasted until May 1945, when the victorious allies restored food supplies. Years later, research workers were able to look back at detailed medical records of the period. The famine affected women and their babies in different ways depending at which stage of pregnancy starvation began.

Women starved in the later months of pregnancy were more likely to give birth to lighter but otherwise normal babies. Women who were not already pregnant when the famine began were at great risk of becoming temporarily infertile until the food supplies were restored. The women who were starved before conception but did manage to conceive or who were starved in very early pregnancy gave birth months after the food shortage had finished, in the autumn/winter of 1945/6. All the stresses of the war had ended months before, yet the numbers of babies stillborn or dying shortly after birth were much increased. These tragic effects were caused around the time of conception. Over the course of just a few months, the reserves of the women had become so depleted that they were at risk.

Eating Well for a Healthy Pregnancy

Even today, in prosperous countries as well as those where famines are regular hazards, there are still plenty of women who are severely undernourished, either because of poverty or because of strict slimming diets* to keep their weight below that which is biologically best for them. The *quality* of food eaten can also affect the development of the unborn child. There is evidence that deficiencies of vitamins and minerals in the mother may be associated with certain forms of handicap (described in Chapter 9) and also with low birth weight. A low birthweight baby is classified as one weighing less than 2500 g (approximately 5½ lb) and it is known that such babies are more likely to have problems with their health than heavier babies. A baby weighing 3500 g (approximately 7¾ lb) is off to a much better start. The commonest causes of low birth weight are maternal malnutrition, ill health and other forms of deprivation. Close spacing of pregnancies can also increase the risk of a low birthweight baby. This is why it is best to leave an interval of at least eighteen months between births, which means waiting nine months or more after the birth of one baby before trying to conceive again.

Nutrition *does* matter – before pregnancy if the woman is to conceive at all and have reserves in readiness for the early months when the baby's vital organs are forming (and when she may not be able to eat properly – due to temporary feelings of nausea, for instance); in later pregnancy when the baby is growing very quickly; and after the birth in the months of breast-feeding to provide the perfect food for the young infant. Healthy, well-nourished mothers – and fathers – have the best chance of having a healthy baby.

Nourishment in its widest sense means more than what you eat; this is why this book deals not only with food, but also touches on smoking and alcohol, drugs and pollutants, exercise and rest, stress and relaxation. The aim is to give practical guidelines (and the reasons for these) before, during and after pregnancy. Such reasons are not intended

---

* The word 'diet' in this book means what you or anyone else eats every day, i.e. one's habitual food. When reference is made to special diets related to losing weight, these will be called 'slimming diets' or 'low-calorie diets'.

It Takes Two

to cause alarm – as noted at the beginning, most babies in the United Kingdom are born normal. Nutrition is but one of a whole host of factors that can influence your health and your life, and that of your baby. Even so, good nutrition can help to swing the balance in favour of you producing the healthiest baby possible.

For men only

Before you invest any money in a house, car or business, make any major decision at work, or prepare to start a repair job on the house, it is likely that you will consider what materials or assets are necessary and how you can ensure the best results. As a father-to-be you may find you are invited – indeed, urged – to attend antenatal classes and prepare yourself for the new arrival. But did you give any consideration to the implications of your life-style even *before* your partner conceived?

When *you* were a baby inside your mother's womb, the cells which would later manufacture sperm were already present in primitive form inside your testes. This means that your potential ability to have children could have been influenced from that time. For the majority of men, from the time of puberty, these special cells act as a continual production line busy in the long and complex process of manufacturing new sperm.

A sperm is one of the tiniest cells of the body but it has the potential to determine the sex of your baby and carry your half of the necessary genetic information. It is also powerful enough to swim a vast distance for its size and overcome all manner of hazards before it reaches its destination – her egg, or ovum. The formation of sperm takes about nine weeks and then a few more weeks are spent in transit down the elongated, coiled tube (the epididymis) attached to the testis and in storage there, awaiting ejaculation. During this period of formation and transport (approximately three months) the cells which produce sperm and the sperm themselves are vulnerable and can be damaged.

The special 'stem' cells which make sperm do, however, have an enormous capacity for recovery. Even if there has been some event or sequence of events which adversely affects your fertility, the 'conveyor belt' system producing sperm can usually return to normal in the following months. If the sperm are damaged, it is generally considered that they will die, be selected out or fail to reach the ovum. However, it is known that on rare occasions such sperm may survive and even fertilize an egg. A varying proportion of the sperm you produce will be misshaped or otherwise abnormal; just how great this proportion is may depend on certain aspects of your life-style, as explained below.

The food you eat
In animal husbandry, special attention is given not only to the nutritional needs of the female but also to those of the male and good diets are fed to breeding stallions, bulls, boars and rams. For you, as a human male, nutrition is especially important during the maturation of your reproductive system in adolescence. After this time, your system is not as sensitive to undernutrition or poor quality food as that of your partner, but it can still be adversely affected by extremes of starvation or poor diet. At the other end of the scale, gross overweight can also affect fertility and depress your sperm count. A good general guide to a healthy weight for your height is the Quetelet index described in Chapter 3. (An index of 20–25 is ideal.)

Good quality food is necessary to supply the nutrients for the maintenance of the testes, the continued production of healthy sperm and the various nutritive secretions which accompany the sperm on its journey after formation. The principles of healthy eating are summarized in Chapter 2 and there are suggestions for further reading should this subject be of particular interest to you.

Smoking – possible consequences
Men who smoke heavily have lower levels of the male hormone testosterone, are more likely to be infertile and may produce a larger proportion of abnormally shaped sperm than non-smoking men. The general view is that such abnormal sperm are selected out. However, the possibility that defects in tiny embryos could be caused by sperm damaged by heavy smoking by the father, cannot be

entirely ruled out. This subject has not yet been widely investigated but one survey in Germany found a very slightly increased risk of the baby dying around the time of birth, associated with heavy smoking by the father, even if the mother was a non-smoker.

Alcohol – possible consequences
It is well known that excessive alcohol intake can cause 'brewer's droop' or temporary impotence in a man. What is not so well known is that regular heavy drinking of alcohol has been linked with poor fertility in men. Furthermore, although it has been assumed for a long time that alcohol presents no genetic hazard (that is, the ability to damage the 'plan' in the sperm), recently this view has been challenged. When alcohol was given to male mice on three consecutive days at certain periods before mating, there was an increased risk that some of the tiny embryos would die in the mother's womb. This raises the possibility that some miscarriages could be attributable to heavy drinking by the father in the weeks or months *before* conception.

Temperature and the testes
The testes are outside the body because they need to be kept at a lower temperature than the rest of the body. Tight jockey pants of synthetic materials such as nylon, and tight trousers, can be constricting and allow the temperature of the scrotum to rise above that which is desirable. If your sperm count is found to be low, you may be advised to wear loose trousers and loose cotton underpants and to avoid taking hot baths or showers.

Diseases and disorders
There are certain infections, for example, adult mumps and venereal disease, and medical disorders such as coeliac disease (a disorder of the digestive system), and diabetes, which can affect a man's fertility and the quality of his sperm. For some, the consequence of such conditions may even be infertility. This could be temporary and treatable (as in the case of coeliacs) or it may be permanent (as it is occasionally following severe adult mumps). A lowered sperm count can be caused by poorly controlled diabetes or

Eating Well for a Healthy Pregnancy

by high blood pressure. Epileptic men may produce more abnormal sperm than average but it is not completely clear whether it is the epilepsy that is damaging or the drugs being taken. Do consult your doctor if you have any queries relating to the possibility that a disease or disorder might affect your reproductive function.

Influence of drugs

Certain drugs have the potential to damage sperm and reduce fertility. Again, it is assumed but not yet proven that such sperm would not normally get through to the ovum and perhaps produce a damaged embryo. The consequences of minor degrees of damage to sperm have not been well documented. If you are in any doubt about any drug you have to take, ask your doctor to check with the manufacturers or with local or national drug information services for details of possible reproductive hazards.

Chemicals and work hazards

Certain industrial chemicals have been reported as having effects on male reproductive function. These include decreased libido or even impotence (for example, caused by chloroprene, vinyl chloride, inorganic mercury) and testicular damage and reduced fertility (for example, caused by kepone, dibromochloropropane, organic lead). There have also been suggestions that some chemicals could cause a reduction in the weight of offspring or increase the risk of miscarriage in the partner. If you and your partner are still at the stage of planning to start a baby or if you have in the past had some problem related to pregnancy and you think you may be exposed to hazards at work, it is worth checking up on these as described in Chapter 5.

Your role during the pregnancy

At conception, your biological input to your son or daughter is complete but you still have a vital role in contributing to your future child's welfare, in terms of giving practical and moral support to your partner during her pregnancy. If she has pregnancy sickness, reading Chapter 6 may give you some ideas on how you can help her to cope. Understanding and tolerance are essential and a

It Takes Two

sense of humour almost as necessary. It is quite common for foods fancied one day to be rejected the next and your kitchen could be stocked up with all manner of odd foods. However, gradually or perhaps even almost overnight, your partner's fads, discomfort or lassitude will disappear and she may find a new lease of energy. If you go out to celebrate on the strength of this or for any other reason, do not encourage her to drink alcohol – and smoking, for her, is taboo. If you both normally smoke, it will help her to abstain if you do not smoke in her presence.

You will soon discover in what ways you can best help during the pregnancy – it may be just a question of doing some of the housework or heavy shopping; it may include acting as an intermediary between your partner and well-meaning but potentially disturbing advisers. Even if you've been through it all before, you may take on some new responsibility, such as catering for the rest of the family while your wife is in hospital. You may already know enough about cooking to be voted chef of the year by the kids but if not, here are a few ideas for simple but nourishing meals.

☐ Cheese-baked eggs. Gently break eggs into a buttered oven-proof dish. Grate some cheese over the top. Cook in oven or under a moderately hot grill. Serve with bread or potatoes and vegetables or salad.

☐ Baked beans on toast with a salad (grated raw carrot with chopped lettuce or grated raw cabbage, cottage cheese and a sprinkling of raisins or currants).

☐ Cold meat with tomatoes and baked potatoes (scrub and clean potatoes, stab each one a few times with a fork to prevent bursting. To reduce cooking time, wrap in foil, impale on skewers and bake on the top shelf in a hot oven). Serve potatoes with butter, cottage cheese or grated hard cheese.

☐ Chicken joints (wrapped in foil they will cook fairly quickly in a moderately hot oven or under the grill), served with spaghetti (quicker to prepare than potatoes) and tomato ketchup, and vegetables.

☐ Bacon with cauliflower and wholemeal bread.

Eating Well for a Healthy Pregnancy

- ☐ Bought fish and chips with some frozen peas.
- ☐ Sausage and mash with cabbage and chutney or ketchup.

If your wife or girlfriend has the baby in hospital, after the birth gifts of food will be most appreciated. Do not take too much at any one time – hospitals are usually very hot and foods can go off quickly in bedside cupboards. If you possess a wide-necked flask, thin sticks of fresh carrot or celery may be welcome, or fill the flask with ice-cubes (to make the lukewarm water she may have to drink more palatable). Other ideas include:

- ☐ A fresh wholemeal roll with butter and her favourite cheese or thinly-sliced cold meat.
- ☐ Crispbreads or cheese biscuits plus a small carton of butter, and honey or cheese – remember to take a knife.
- ☐ A carton of yogurt and a spoon.
- ☐ Small pack of nuts and raisins.
- ☐ Fresh fruit.

Once back at home, it will soon become obvious that your new baby can create work out of all proportion to his or her size. You may both feel tired and drained in the early weeks and it is important to look after yourself as well as your partner. Ten minutes snooze in the lunch hour may do you more good than a strong cup of coffee to keep awake during the afternoon. Eat regular meals even if you do have to help to make them. Life will begin to settle down into some sort of pattern quite soon.

Over the coming months and years, there will be many things which have the potential to affect the long-term wellbeing of your son or daughter. Of those factors which you can influence, good nutrition is one which is of paramount importance.

TWO

Healthy Eating

When you start to be interested in what you eat, you soon find there is no shortage of information, though it is often more about what *not* to eat rather than what is good for you. Angela was eager to have a healthy baby and resolved to cut down on 'junk' food and change her erratic eating habits. Little did she realize what was in store when she sought advice from doctor, midwife, mother and friends. They all seemed to have very fixed, but contradictory, views. Who could be right? To confuse matters further, it seemed that every week in the newspaper, yet another food was reported to be 'bad' for health, while advertising on TV and in magazines showed men and women apparently brimful of health and vitality consuming the latest soft drink, 'instant' soup, or chocolate snack – the very items she had given up!

This book is intended for anyone who, like Angela, is interested in good health and wants basic guidelines on healthy eating but does not want to be tied to calorie-counters or menu sheets. These guidelines are relevant not only to pregnancy but also to lifelong eating habits.

Healthy eating *can* be simple. You do not need a nutrition textbook or a book of food tables; just a modicum of common sense and a willingness to go right back to fundamental principles when choosing what to eat. Try to imagine what you would do if you had just arrived on earth and were totally ignorant of all the information which had been written about food. People you saw shopping might be choosing food for reasons far removed from health and more related to appearance, colour, the influence of TV advertising or special offers. To find out what was healthy, you would probably try to find some healthy people and take note of what they were eating, rather than spend your time looking at what unhealthy people were eating.

Studies *have* been made – some conducted earlier this

century – of the eating habits of healthy societies. Note has also been made of the health problems which develop when eating habits change with the introduction of modern foods such as white flour and sugar. Although some research workers became convinced that this or that particular type of diet was *the right one* for health, it has gradually become apparent that there is no single healthy diet; there are many possible healthy alternatives. The healthy Hunza people of northern India, for example ate a largely lactovegetarian diet of wheat and other grains, green and root vegetables, fruit, pulses, milk, butter and cheese, with meat on occasions. Equally healthy, however, were the islanders of the Faroes, Iceland, and Greenland, who were almost entirely carnivorous – eating an animal, bird or fish diet. Still different combinations of foods were eaten by other healthy groups of people.

Some may argue that these studies just proved that exactly what you eat cannot be so very important to health and, certainly, the types of food, the climate and methods of food preparation were very varied. The main conclusion from these studies, however, is not how all the eating patterns *differed*, but in what ways they were *similar*. Some fundamental principles were common to them all.

These healthy diets were *whole*, that is, there were no highly refined foods such as white bread, sugar and soft drinks. When bread was eaten it contained most or all of the wheat grain. On many occasions the whole of the fruit or vegetable was used. Eating meat meant eating a wide variety of the edible parts of the carcass, including what we call offal (liver, kidneys, brains, heart, etc) and the muscle meat and skin. Even the bones were made into stock. For some people, sadly, the words 'whole' or 'wholesome' conjure up images of health food shops or 'crank' diets, which for some reason they think they should avoid. Whole foods are not special foods, only foods which have not been highly refined. Wholemeal bread is a whole food but so too is a whole sardine, a potato baked in its jacket, an apple or a glass of whole milk.

These people ate plenty of *fresh* food whenever they could, although they had to depend on stored food at certain times of the year. Today, methods of preservation

Healthy Eating

and refrigeration are highly developed but there is often a price to pay in loss of nutrients. This does not matter if fresh food is eaten most of the time, but it has become possible to get through a whole day without eating any fresh food at all. For reasons of convenience, many people rely on dried milk for drinks, tinned or frozen vegetables, preserved and packet meats – even when fresh seasonal foods may be no more expensive or even cheaper. Yet it *is* important to include fresh foods in your daily diet.

For the people in the studies mentioned, *simple food preparation* and processing ensured maximum preservation of food value. Their nutritional status was not put in jeopardy by overconsumption of highly processed but nutritionally inferior dried and instant foods with long lists of ingredients, flavourings, colours, preservatives and other non-food ingredients, such as are readily available today.

The good quality of their food was ensured by the *cycle* of nutrients between man, animals, plants and the soil or sea. This was achieved either by nature alone or by careful agricultural methods which respected nature's laws. Today's pristine clean and plastic-wrapped food can seem far removed from nature even though its quality still depends ultimately on the soil or sea. Modern farming methods which remove crop after crop and replace only a few selected nutrients in the form of chemical fertilizers must lead to a gradual decline in soil and crop health. Unhealthy crops are more susceptible to fungal and insect attack, and this in turn can lead to the application of even more chemicals to combat disease.

Most of us can do very little about this. For the foreseeable future, the bulk of our food will come from 'conventional' farming methods. However, we do have available today many different foods from all over the world so we can compensate for possible inferiority of quality by eating a wide variety of foods.

If you do have the time to grow some of your own food 'organically' or if you can afford it and are lucky enough to have access to organically grown food, whether it be free range eggs, meat and poultry, vegetables and fruit, or wholemeal flour and cereals, then they are worth the extra cost and effort involved.

Eating Well for a Healthy Pregnancy

Your own healthy eating plan

Wherever you shop, be it supermarket or village shop, and whatever the size of your kitchen and purse, you can develop your own healthy eating plan by following these basic principles:

1 *Eat whole foods* – wholemeal bread and wholegrain cereals, whole vegetables and fruits when appropriate, and a range of animal foods which include more than just muscle meats.

2 *Eat some fresh foods daily*, for example, fresh milk and fresh vegetables, both raw in salads and cooked.

3 *Keep food preparation simple* most of the time and, as often as you can, prepare your own menus and recipes starting with basic ingredients.

4 *Choose a wide variety of foods.* Unless your diet is limited for religious or moral reasons or because of some allergy or medical condition, a varied well-balanced diet will supply all the nutrients you need. One simple way of choosing a well-balanced diet from the vast array of foods available so that you will get the right balance of nutrients, is to divide foods up into four groups.

These groups are:

1 Meat and alternatives.
2 Bread and cereals.
3 Vegetables and fruit.
4 Milk and milk products.

Some traditional meals are well-balanced mixes from these groups, for example:

Roast beef (meat group), and Yorkshire pudding (cereal group and milk group), plus potatoes and greens (vegetable group).
Pizza has a bread base (cereal group) and a small amount of fish or meat (meat group), plus tomatoes (vegetable group) and cheese topping (milk group).

An example of a vegetarian dish is:
Bean and vegetable casserole (beans come from the meat

Healthy Eating

and alternatives group, together with the vegetable group) served with wholemeal bread (cereal group) and cheese or yogurt (milk group).

The four food groups are illustrated in the diagram below and described in more detail in the text which follows.

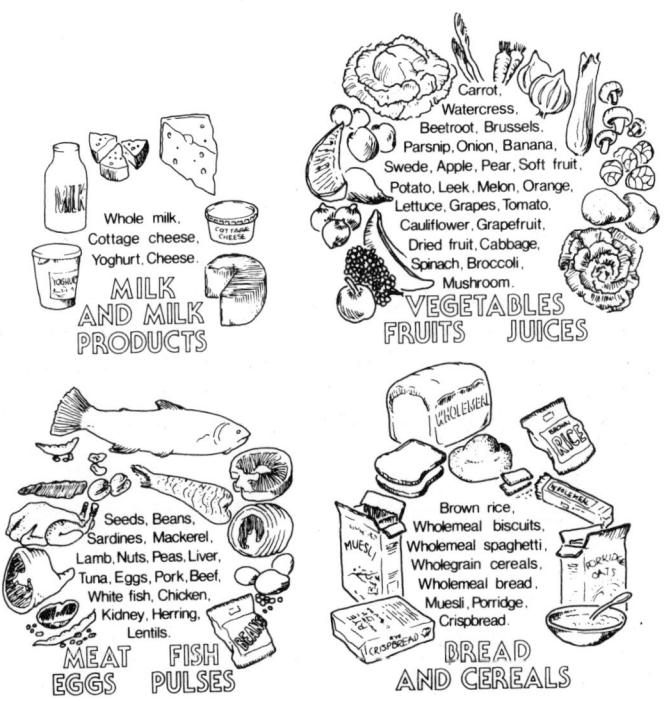

1 Meat and alternatives

This group contains both animal and vegetable foods which are good sources of protein. Those people who are mainly 'carnivorous' and those who are strictly vegan are in the minority. Between these two extremes are the majority who have the option to pick and choose right across the spectrum of animal and vegetable proteins – meat, fish, poultry, eggs, pulses, nuts and seeds.

If you are a meat eater, choose a wide range of meats. Include 'offal', which means the organ meats: liver, kidney, brains, tongue, sweetbreads, and heart. These are especially good for pregnancy as they are a rich source of many vitamins and minerals. Try to eat liver once a week. (If you are worried about toxins in liver, eat lamb's liver as most lambs are not reared intensively or on heavily fertilized pasture.) Brains, like liver, are rich in the essential but often neglected 'structural' fats (as opposed to the 'storage' fat found in and around muscle). Heart contains very little extra fat and waste and is very tasty in a stew or stuffed. If you find kidneys too strong by themselves try them in steak and kidney pudding or pie.

Muscle meats vary a great deal in price, depending on demand and on tenderness. However, in terms of nutritional value, stewing beef is as good as best steak and sometimes joints can work out as better value than quicker cooking chops. Trotters and bones make excellent stock for soup and it is worth obtaining marrow bones to make marrow stock for baby soups during weaning.

Chicken and even turkey, once more expensive than meat, are now relatively cheap as a result of factory farming methods. If available, free-range or older birds can be more tasty than broilers but may need more cooking. Poultry carcasses make excellent 'white' stock for soups and sauces. Duck, pheasant, guinea fowl and grouse are worth keeping in mind for special occasions. A pheasant usually has far more meat on it than a larger-looking duck. Rabbit is also classed as game but is often cheap enough for regular use in pies, stews or curries.

The institution of 'fish on Friday' for religious reasons had the bonus of being nutritionally sound. Once, or better still, twice a week, eat fish – both white and oily. Fish varies a lot in price and, as with meat, the dearest is not necessarily the best from a health point of view. Cod and coley are cheaper white fish than halibut or plaice. Oily fish – including herring, mackerel, sprats, sardines, tuna and pilchards as well as the more expensive trout and salmon – are richer sources of many different nutrients than white fish.

The egg is a high quality animal food and a real 'whole' food – it contains everything necessary for a chick to grow. It is a mistaken view to think that eggs may be harmful –

Healthy Eating

they can form a significant part of a well-balanced diet and are an especially valuable food for pregnancy since they contain a wide range of vitamins and minerals.

Other alternatives to meat and fish are the 'pulses' – peas, beans and lentils. Apart from green peas and baked beans, both undoubtedly good foods, there are many other pulses – for example, split peas, black-eyed beans, chick peas, haricot beans (which make baked beans), lentils, mung beans, kidney beans, butter beans, and soyabeans. Health food shops and some supermarkets and grocers offer a range of these and also of the many foods made from soyabeans such as tofu (soyabean curd), tempeh (fermented soyabean curd), miso (soyabean paste), as well as soy flour and soy milk. Plant proteins add further variety to your diet and are much cheaper sources of protein than meat.

Nuts and seeds can boost the protein content of a meal containing only a little meat, for example used in a side salad or as part of a dessert. Other uses are in home baking, as the basis of a vegetarian main course, in stuffings or as snacks. Many of us are familiar with almonds, brazils, walnuts and hazelnuts at Christmas time. These and many others, such as pistachios, cashews and pecans, are now widely available (ready shelled) throughout the year. They are on sale in a few supermarkets as well as in health food shops and good grocers. The peanut really belongs to the pulse family – it is a ground bean or 'pea' nut. Peanut butter can be used as a sandwich spread or in various vegetarian dishes; there are many brands available and some do not contain added sugar and salt.

Sunflower and ground sesame seeds are just two of the edible seeds available. Their main use is as a garnish or flavouring for breads and salads, as a toasted topping, in casseroles, muesli, and stuffings or ground to be used as spreads.

The above list of foods is just a guide to the wide range of meat and alternatives available – not an instruction manual. Eat what you are happy with. There is no point in forcing yourself to eat either soyapaste or peanut butter if you cannot stand the taste or the texture, or a lamb chop if even the sight of it makes you shudder. Nor does your eating plan have to be *either* animal *or* vegetable protein. Even

Eating Well for a Healthy Pregnancy

within one meal, many delicious dishes are a combination of animal and vegetable foods, and were often originally developed as a means of extending a scarce or expensive meat protein. For those who are not wholly vegetarian, vegetarian dishes can be very useful for lunch or supper, whichever is not the main meal, for example:

Beans on toast.
Vegetables with rice.
Macaroni cheese.
Bean and vegetable soups.
Fruit and nut breads.

2 Bread and cereals

The grain of wheat contains all the nutrients for the early development of a new plant, yet over hundreds of years it has become customary for millers to spend more and more time and effort removing the outer coat of the grain (bran) and the growing point (germ) which is the most nutritious part of all. The flour made from the remaining white starchy centre (which the millers like because it keeps better than wholemeal flour and has a very smooth texture) is used to make the modern white loaf. White bread is 'fortified' which means that a few vitamins and minerals are added but this 'fortification' is merely a token effort to compensate for a whole host of nutrients damaged or lost by removal of the bran and germ. Because wholemeal bread contains more vitamins and minerals than white, it is a better buy for pregnancy. If you want wholemeal, read the label or ask; many so-called 'brown' and 'wheatmeal' breads actually contain a large proportion of white flour.

Wheat is just one of the many 'cereal' grains. Others are oats, rye, barley, millet, rice, maize and buckwheat. For variety try the dark continental rye-breads, wholemeal versions of Greek pitta bread and the many types of homemade breads. Hardbreads or crispbread add even more variety and are useful to serve with cheese as a dessert or for a snack. There are crunchy wholegrain crispbreads, not to be confused with some of the starch-reduced slimmers' crispbreads, and biscuits such as oatcakes. Digestives, 'bran' biscuits and other types of wheatmeal biscuits usually contain a mixture of refined and

Healthy Eating

wholemeal flours together with added bran, and some are sweetened.

The traditional way to enjoy 'cereal' is as a breakfast food. The least processed and most wholesome breakfast cereals are oatmeal and rolled oats, used for porridge or muesli. Oats are a very cheap cereal. Many of the readymade mueslis are expensive and some contain a lot of sugar. It is cheaper to buy a muesli base containing flakes of oats and of other grains such as barley, rye and wheat, or buy all the flakes separately and mix them yourself. To this base you can add whatever you like – chopped or ground nuts, dried fruit, fresh apple, banana and so on.

Some of the packet cereals are based on the wholegrain, e.g. shredded wheat and wheat biscuit types. Many others are highly refined, highly processed and contain a lot of sugar as well as flavourings, colour and other additives, and they can work out very expensive in relation to nutritional content. Shop with a critical eye and always read the labels carefully. Then you will not be deceived by pictures or words chosen to conjure up a 'healthy' rustic image nor by impressive looking lists of vitamins and minerals which are usually added in an attempt to compensate for nutrients removed during processing.

Rice and pasta are cereals which are the staple foods in many countries. Depending on price and preference, use these as part of your daily, weekly or monthly choice of cereals. Apply the 'wholesome' principle, though in some areas finding wholemeal pasta and brown rice might be difficult. If they are not on sale in your local shop or supermarket, try asking for them. The management usually likes to please customers and some supermarkets already stock wholemeal spaghetti.

3 Vegetables and fruit

The wide variety of fresh produce displayed on open market stalls or in greengrocers is very much a part of the British way of life, yet it is often neglected by many people. This is unfortunate because vegetables and fruit have a long established reputation for being good sources of many vitamins, minerals, certain essential oils and fibre. However, there are differences among the various vegetables and

Eating Well for a Healthy Pregnancy

fruits not only in taste but in nutrient content. Some are good sources of vitamin C, some of the B vitamin called folate, and some of a substance called carotene which is a forerunner of another vitamin, vitamin A. Because of these differences, fruit and vegetables are often subdivided into three categories which relate to vitamin content. Taking some from each group daily before, during and after pregnancy will ensure the right mix of vitamins. The categories are:

☐ *Vitamin C-rich fruit and vegetables*
Citrus fruits and juices; grapefruit, orange, tangerine and lemon.
Strawberries, raspberries, blackberries, blackcurrants, melon.
Potatoes (vitamin C content differs greatly and declines during winter).
Tomatoes, watercress, peppers, mustard and cress.
Cabbage, Brussels sprouts, broccoli, cauliflower, spring 'greens'.

☐ *Leafy green vegetables and fruits which contain folate* (many of these are also rich sources of carotene)
Broccoli, Brussels sprouts, cabbage.
Dark leafy lettuce, endive, watercress.
Spinach, kale, beet tops.
Oranges, pineapple, dates, avocado, nectarines, and cantaloupe melon.

☐ *Other fruits and vegetables*
Carrot, turnip, swede, parsnip, potato, radish, beetroot.
French and runner beans, sugar peas, sweetcorn, peas.
Onions, lettuce, beansprouts, mushrooms, cucumber, celery, cauliflower.
Apricots, nectarines, peaches, watermelon, plum.
Apple, pear, cherries, berries, grapes, banana, pineapple.
Prunes, dates, figs, raisins, sultanas, currants.

Be liberal in your use of vegetables: eat them every day both cooked and raw, perhaps as a salad – either with your lunch or as a side salad with an evening meal. It need not be exotic, just use whatever is cheap, fresh and seasonal. Vegetables are one item of your diet which should not be neglected.

Healthy Eating

When fruit is expensive eat more vegetables instead – a main meal could be meat or alternatives with three portions of vegetables rather than two portions of vegetables and then one of fruit. Try to include some citrus fruit daily – whole and fresh whenever possible or pure unsweetened juices when the whole fruit is expensive. Fresh fruit is best but canned and frozen fruits are useful occasionally; for example, pineapple canned in its own juice is widely available. Some other canned fruits can now be obtained in their own juice. Fruits such as raspberries, frozen at the peak of the season, can give a touch of summer to desserts later in the year.

Dried fruits are good sources of many minerals but lack vitamin C, which is removed during the drying process. Raisins, sultanas and dates can all be used in salads, snacks, muesli, and fruit cakes. Other dried fruits include prunes, apricots, figs, peaches, fruit salad, and even bananas. For vegetarians dried fruit can contribute significantly to iron needs.

4 Milk and milk products

These foods are particularly good for pregnancy as they contain so many different nutrients: protein, carbohydrate, fat, vitamins and minerals, and especially calcium. The calcium in milk is readily available to the human body and this makes it valuable for meeting the increased need for calcium during pregnancy and lactation.

A tiny minority of people need to avoid milk because they are allergic or lactose-intolerant, but for most of us milk is an excellent food for pregnancy and for babies after weaning.

Buy milk whole, not skimmed, and as fresh as you can get it, which usually means pasteurized. Skimmed milk can cost more and has lost nutritional value; it is not recommended for pregnant women or babies in their first year (it was tried unsuccessfully in Canada). Sterilized, ultra-heat treated (UHT), and dried milks are more highly processed than pasteurized. The best milk of all to buy is 'Green Top', or untreated milk – sadly, only available in a few areas. Official testing nowadays is very efficient and, providing the milk comes from a reliable and hygienic source, untreated milk is far superior in all respects – taste, nutritional value, and ability to 'keep' – than pasteurized, UHT or sterilized. Goat milk, also untreated, is becoming increasingly popular and is a good buy under certain conditions – *if* you can get it, *if* you can afford it, *if* it is produced hygienically, and *if* it is very fresh (or frozen soon after milking) as it soon develops 'off' flavours.

One pint of milk (or milk plus yogurt) a day should be a minimum during pregnancy and breast-feeding. If you really cannot drink milk (as distinct from thinking you should not), try natural yogurt instead, either by itself, with fruit or fruit purée, in salad dressings, soups, muesli or with main dishes such as stews and curries.

Good cheese can be expensive but has more flavour and value than the more highly processed but cheaper alternatives. The best cheeses are the 'farmhouse' varieties of English cheese such as Cheddar and Cheshire (there are at least nine other varieties) and some of the continental ones. To make good cheese needs good milk; the current restrictions on antibiotics in milk – designed originally not so much to protect the consumer as the cheese industry – are severe. Antibiotics in milk would detrimentally affect the cheese-making process. Cheese is an important food as part of a varied diet but a lot of it is not a good substitute for milk. Why? There are two groups of protein in milk – the casein and the whey – both are good for health but the whey, which is best, is lost during the cheese-making process. Some of the water soluble vitamins are lost too. Cottage cheese has a lower content of some vitamins, such as vitamin B_6, than hard cheese but it has many uses, both in savoury and sweet dishes.

Cream is a very good, rich food, best reserved for its traditional use with a fruit dessert or as an addition to soup. Butter is a natural product, made simply by churning cream and adding a little salt. No artificial flavourings or preservatives are added. Cream and butter are made from milk but are *not* included in the milk group when you are counting serving sizes, because they are used only in small amounts. Together with other fats and oils, use these as 'extras' to the mixture of basic foods which you take from the four groups.

Opinions about the value of milk, butter, and cream have

Healthy Eating

changed dramatically over the last fifty years. They have long been high on the list of foods good for health, so why is there such a strong anti-milk lobby today? Sadly, it is because desperate attempts have been made to single out just one 'villain' to answer for such problems as heart disease and allergy. In fact, it is far more likely that a whole complex of dietary and environmental factors are responsible. There is no evidence that milk and dairy products, as part of a wholesome diet, are in any way harmful during pregnancy or in the long-term, for the majority of people. However, this information does not receive the publicity it deserves. Most, but not all, margarines are highly processed, contain colouring, flavouring, and other additives such as antioxidants, emulsifiers, stabilizers and preservatives and are at last coming under suspicion for possible harmful effects. If you are vegan or prefer to use margarine, go for the best quality margarines (usually indicated by a higher price).

A well-balanced diet for pregnancy

There are people who weigh or measure their food precisely and pore over complicated charts trying to work out what to eat, but such dedication and accuracy is not necessary for the maintenance of health. Providing you are moderately physically active every day, eat unrefined foods, and choose a wide range of foods (for example, by using the four food group scheme described) then your body will be your best guide as to when and how much to eat.

Because individuals vary enormously in their nutritional needs - for reasons of age, build, height, metabolic rate and so on - it is impossible to state categorically that you would need so many calories before or during pregnancy, and so much fat, protein, carbohydrates, vitamins and minerals etc. Some books do stipulate in quite a detailed way the quantities of foods required during pregnancy, but these recommendations differ from book to book! The chart overleaf is intended as a very general guide to the number of portions from each group which could make up a well-balanced diet for pregnancy.

Eating Well for a Healthy Pregnancy

- *Meat and alternatives* If you take large portions, e.g. two eggs, 4 oz cooked meat, 5 oz cooked fish, two portions from this group is ample.

  If you take medium portions, e.g. 1 egg, 2–3 oz meat, fish or poultry, 1 cup of beans, peas or lentils, three portions daily will be enough.

  If you take small or even tiny portions, such as small amounts of nuts, peas, beans, or meat (1–2 oz), then you will need to take sufficient portions so that, when added together, they make up the equivalent of two large portions.

  If you are vegetarian, 1 cup of beans, peas or lentils, plus 3 tablespoons of nuts or seeds, plus 1 egg will be enough (when combined with the milk group and extra servings of cereals).

  If you are vegan, see Chapter 7.

- *Bread and cereals* Five portions daily (6–7 in a vegetarian menu). For example, one portion could be a bowl of cereal, or one slice of wholemeal bread, or a helping of brown rice or of pasta.

- *Vegetables and fruit* Five or more portions. Include at least 2 vitamin C-rich vegetables and fruit, 2 in the leafy green folate-rich group and 1 other fruit or vegetable. (These groups have been described in the previous section).

- *Milk and milk products* Three to four portions. Preferably this should include 1 pint of milk (which might represent two to three portions, depending on appetite, e.g. 1 portion on cereal and 1 large or 2 small glasses of milk. A carton of yogurt or a piece of cheese (e.g. 1½ oz) would also be equivalent to a portion).

- *Fats and oils* These are classed as extras to the food groups and usually 1–2 tablespoons (1–2 oz) are recommended, depending on needs.

These numbers of servings should be regarded as baseline minimums, from which to add, depending on your body size and appetite. They should be increased if you are underweight, physically very active, carrying twins, or have had some serious problem with a previous pregnancy. If you have a medical condition which may require a modified diet

Healthy Eating

or if you have special problems or queries relating to your diet, ask your doctor about the possibility of seeing a dietitian or request to see the dietitian at your antenatal clinic.

What about your needs before pregnancy and after the birth? As a guide only, *before pregnancy* you may find yourself eating one portion *less* from each of the milk and the cereal groups. *After pregnancy*, when you are breast-feeding, you may need to add one portion *more* from each of the milk and the cereal groups.

The tables on pages 28–32 give an example of this basic diet (X) together with a breakdown of the various foods into the groups detailed above and more detailed information on specific nutrients. For comparative purposes, another sample diet (Y), is shown; it can be seen that this contains a great deal less of certain nutrients than diet X. The nutrients marked * are those which fall below the current UK or American standards for pregnancy.

Does this eating plan fulfil needs for calories, protein, carbohydrate, fat, vitamins and minerals?

Calories. The number of calories in the example given is less than current recommendations for pregnancy but it approximates more closely to what dietary surveys have found that pregnant women actually eat. Obviously, if you need more calories because you are, for instance, tall or very active, then you will feel hungrier and eat more.

Protein. The amount of protein needed for good health during pregnancy has become a much debated issue. At one extreme are those who believe that no extra protein at all is needed over and above your non-pregnant needs and at the other are those who press for a large protein intake. Who is right? Those who argue that no extra protein is required may be right but only with two very important provisos:

1. That the woman's diet is already adequate in protein.
2. That she is taking enough carbohydrate and fat to meet her demands for energy.

If these needs are not fulfilled, valuable protein may be used

Eating Well for a Healthy Pregnancy

as an energy source, rather than going towards building the baby's new tissues. Those who argue for an ample protein intake are probably on safer ground – this will ensure adequate protein for the baby's needs and any surplus can be used for the normal energy needs of the mother. Excessive protein is, however, to be avoided as it is wasteful and is of no benefit to your health.

Comparison of two daily diets and their nutrient contents

Diet X	*Diet Y*
1 orange, muesli (oats, nuts, wheatgerm, raisins), boiled egg, 1 slice wholemeal bread with butter, cup of tea. ⅓ pint milk on cereal and in tea.	Cornflakes, 1 tsp sugar, 1 slice white bread and marmalade, 1 mug of coffee with 1 tsp dried milk and 1 tsp sugar, ⅓ pint skimmed milk on cereal.
Weak coffee with milk. Oatcake.	Coffee with 1 tsp dried milk, 1 tsp sugar, 2 semi-sweet biscuits.
2 slices wholemeal bread and butter with ½ tin sardines in tomato sauce, large raw carrot, watercress, apple, glass of milk.	2 slices white bread and margarine, fish paste, packet of crisps, wrapped chocolate biscuit, can of cola.
2 rye crispbread with butter and yeast extract, cup of tea with milk.	2 cream crackers and margarine, jam, cup of tea with 1 tsp dried milk and 1 tsp sugar.
Mince and onions, 2 jacket potatoes, Brussels sprouts, natural yogurt and pear.	Luncheon meat, instant mash, tinned carrot, lemon meringue pie.
Snacks: a few nuts and raisins, glass of milk at bedtime, 1 banana.	Snacks: boiled sweets, cup of tea with 1 tsp dried milk and 1 tsp sugar.

See page 32 for the weights of food used for these two examples.

How many portions of the food groups do these two diets provide?

Meat and alternatives

1 egg, hazelnuts (in muesli and snack), sardine and mince.	Fish paste, luncheon meat, tiny amount of egg in lemon meringue pie.

Healthy Eating

These satisfy the need for 2 large or 4 small portions and supply enough protein.	These do not meet the need for protein (see list of nutrients).

Bread and cereals

Oats and wheatgerm, 3 slices wholemeal bread, rye crispbread, and oatcake.	Cornflakes, 3 slices of white bread, cream crackers, biscuits, chocolate biscuit, pastry in pie.
These satisfy the need for 5 portions.	These satisfy the need for number of portions but the highly refined foods do not meet the need for vitamins and minerals.

Vegetables and fruit

Orange, potato – 2 vitamin C sources. Brussels sprouts, watercress – 2 leafy green sources. Banana, onion, pear, carrot – other vegetables and fruit.	Instant mash – 1 vitamin C source. Lemon (in pie) – a vitamin C source?? Crisps, carrot – other veg.
These satisfy the need for 5 or more portions.	These do not meet the need for vegetables and fruit. There are no leafy green vegetables. This means the diet is inadequate in vitamin C and folate.

Milk and milk products

1 pint milk = 3 portions. Natural yogurt.	Skimmed milk – ⅓ pint. Dried milk – 4 tsp.
These satisfy the need for 3–4 portions.	These do not satisfy the need for 3–4 portions.

Fats and oils

Butter	Margarine.

Miscellaneous

Yeast extract.	Sugar, sweets, marmalade, jam, cola drinks. These supply little besides calories.

Eating Well for a Healthy Pregnancy

	Diet X	Diet Y
Calories	2220*	2228*
Protein (g)	102	54*
Fat (g)	88	90
Unsaturated fat (g)	41	22
Carbohydrate (g)	273	321
Fibre (g)	40	19
Vitamins		
Vitamin A (µg)	2677	1045
Vitamin D (µg)	5.8****	3.1****
Vitamin E (mg)	10.4	6.1
Vitamin B_1 (mg)	2.0	1.2
Vitamin B_2 (mg)	3.4	1.6
Niacin (mg)	21	15*
Vitamin B_6 (mg)	2.7	0.8**
Vitamin B_{12} (µg)	12.8	2.0*
Pantothenic acid (mg)	7.5	2.8
Folate (µg)	446	72***
Biotin (µg)	53	14
Vitamin C (mg)	158	22***
Minerals		
Calcium (mg)	1584	876
Phosphorus (mg)	2333	1069
Magnesium (mg)	551	167**
Iron (mg)	19.5	10.0**
Zinc (mg)	17.9*	6.3***
Copper (mg)	2.3	1.1

Notes:
- * Nutrients marked thus fall just below the current UK or USA standards.
- ** and *** Nutrients marked thus fall a long way below recommendations.
- **** Vitamin D comes also from sunlight to make up the need for this nutrient.

See page 32 for the amounts of food used for these calculations.

Healthy Eating

The blocks below show the proportions of vitamins and minerals in diet Y 🗒 relative to diet X ☐

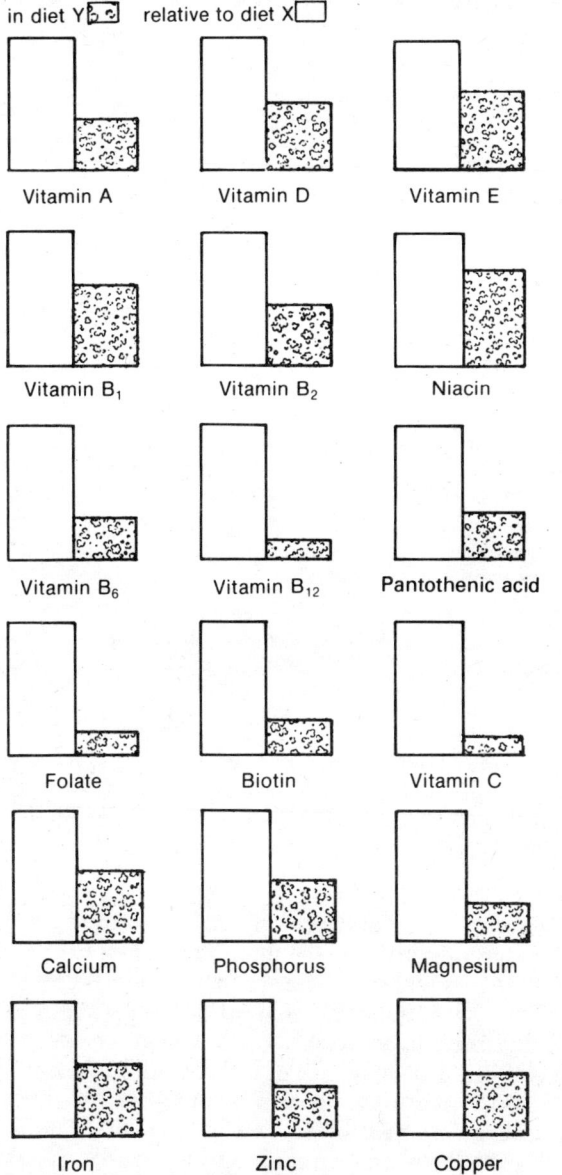

Eating Well for a Healthy Pregnancy

Weights of food used for the calculation of nutrients in diets X and Y

Diet X		*Diet Y*	
Mince	85 g	Luncheon meat	85 g
Boiled egg	60 g	Fish paste	25 g
½ tin of sardines	60 g	Cornflakes	30 g
Hazelnuts	15 g	White bread	100 g
Bread	100 g	Semi-sweet biscuits	20 g
Oats	50 g	Chocolate biscuit	30 g
2 crispbreads	20 g	Cream crackers	20 g
Oatcake	20 g	Lemon meringue pie	120 g
Wheatgerm	10 g	⅓ pint of skimmed milk	190 g
1 pint of milk	568 g	Dried milk	20 g
1 natural yogurt	150 g		
2 jacket potatoes	250 g	Instant mash	150 g
Carrot	100 g	Tinned carrot	60 g
Watercress	20 g	Crisps	25 g
Apple	120 g	Sugar	25 g
Onions	60 g	Marmalade	5 g
Brussels sprouts	112 g	Jam	5 g
Pear	120 g	Sweets	10 g
Orange	120 g	Cola drinks	330 g
Raisins	20 g	Margarine	25 g
Yeast extract	5 g		

Note: These weights are only examples and are not intended as guidelines. If you are tiny and have a sedentary occupation you may eat less than this. Conversely, if you are active or tall and heavy, you may eat more.

A moderate portion of the meat and alternatives group at all meals, together with the recommended amounts of milk, bread and cereals will supply more than enough protein. As can be seen from the table, diet X contains about 100 g protein, an amount associated with a healthy pregnancy and linked with a good intake of the vitamins and minerals present in the various protein sources. Your diet for pregnancy can be a healthy one with less protein than this (60–70 g is thought to be enough by some authorities) but do not err on the side of too little. You know your own body better than anyone else, so respond to its signals. If you feel like eating more fish, eggs, meat, etc at a particular time then do so. Often women go off meat and other protein-rich foods in early pregnancy, then later develop a greater desire for them; while other women, such as vegetarians or those accustomed to a low protein diet before pregnancy, may report feeling an increased craving for protein-rich foods in early pregnancy and sometimes for foods they don't normally consume.

Carbohydrate. Many people hold the mistaken belief that carbohydrate is 'fattening'. Certainly, refined carbohydrates in large amounts are damaging to health – white bread, white sugar, foods made with white flour, confectionery and soft drinks. But unrefined carbohydrate foods – wholemeal bread, cereals, pasta, rice, potatoes and other starchy vegetables and fruits – are good sources not only of energy but of fibre and many other nutrients.

Fat. You may have heard or read about the need to cut down on the amount of fat in your diet. If you have been eating an excessive amount of fried foods and/or a lot of readymade snack foods rich in processed fat (for example, crisps, savoury biscuits and snacks, salted and roasted nuts), by all means cut these right down or cut them out completely.

However, fat is not a forbidden food – we all need it. What is not so well known is that there are two types of fat – the familiar 'storage' fats (like that on a lamb chop or on your own hips) and the not so familiar 'structural' fats, which are absolutely essential as they are contained in every cell and are particularly important constituents of organs such as the brain, liver, kidney and heart.

Where do we get these structural fats from? Some of them can be made in the body from smaller components but others, the essential fatty acids, must come readymade in foods. Both leaves and seeds such as grains and nuts contain these essential fats, as do the oils derived from plant sources. Since animals eat plants, when we eat animal foods, we also eat these fats – providing they have not been lost during food processing. To get enough of these important fats, eat dark green leafy vegetables, food from wholegrains such as the wholemeal bread and other cereals recommended, nuts, fresh (not processed) meat, fish and offal such as liver and brains. By eating according to the plan already described, you will satisfy your needs for these special fats.

Although these needs can be met by choosing food from the four food groups, most people take extra fats and/or oils with their food. This is why an allowance of 1-2 tablespoons is listed after the food groups. Such additional fats might include butter, cream, oil, dripping, lard, and pure vegetable and seed oils (for example, corn oil, sunflower oil and olive oil) rather than blended oils and fats. As well as making food appetizing to eat, fats are good sources of energy when extra calories are needed, they contain vitamins, and they help to produce a feeling of fullness. They can be used in a variety of ways – butter on bread, olive or corn oil for preliminary frying of vegetables in preparation for casseroles and soups, a little cream in soup or on fruit, and sunflower oil for salad dressings.

There is nothing wrong with eating fats and oils but it is essential to keep them in balance with the rest of your diet. If you eat plenty of bread with your butter, lots of salad with the dressing and a good helping of fruit with the cream, your diet will be a healthy one but if you overindulge in fats so they are out of proportion to other nutrients, your health may suffer. Fats and oils and fatty foods are very high in calories and should be treated as luxuries (unless you are climbing a mountain or doing very strenuous work!). For people who are overweight, added fats such as butter, lard, cream and oil should be kept to a minimum because of their very high calorie content but they should not be eliminated entirely. Also, foods which are good sources of the 'structural' fats are still essential.

Fats easily go rancid and the structural fats can be damaged during food processing. The less the interference by manufacturers and processors, the more likely it is that the essential fats will not be lost or damaged. Avoid fats and oils which have been highly processed and/or contain a lot of additives.

Healthy Eating

Vitamins and minerals. These will be adequately supplied if you follow the dietary guidelines suggested and if you also take care to conserve these nutrients when you store and prepare foods at home (see Chapter 4). If you look again at the table on page 30 you will see the different amounts of vitamins and minerals supplied by the two daily diets X and Y. The more highly refined and processed foods are poorer sources of these nutrients. If you are interested in more detailed information about vitamins and minerals, see Chapter 9.

What about other items of diet?

Drinks. How much you need to drink varies enormously depending on your level of activity, the time of year and the stage of pregnancy or breast-feeding. At certain times, you may feel more thirsty than others, so drink as much as you feel you need to satisfy your thirst.

What should you drink? Try to limit tea and coffee drinking to a total of 5 mugs a day or less. Water, milk, pure unsweetened fruit and vegetable juices, and mild herb teas are good alternatives. The range of pure juices widely available now includes apple and grape juice in addition to grapefruit, pineapple and orange. Dilute these for a long drink or, if you are fond of fizzy drinks, add plain soda water or a naturally sparkling mineral water to the pure juice. These are better for you than large amounts of soft drinks such as cola and lemonade. Alcohol should be avoided or restricted to occasional use; a discussion of the reasons why is given in Chapter 5.

Salt. Most people consume considerably more salt than they need and great efforts are now being made to encourage people to cut down on the salt they add to foods during cooking and on the many readymade, liberally salted foods such as crisps and salted nuts. However, in the past enthusiastic efforts to restrict the intake of salt by pregnant women had unfortunate consequences and it is now realized that a pregnant woman may actually need *more* salt than usual. This does not mean that you should purposefully add extra salt; rather that you should *not* try to

Eating Well for a Healthy Pregnancy

restrict it – just salt your food according to taste. If you have some special disorder for which your salt intake has to be carefully restricted, seek medical advice.

Herbs and spices. Besides adding variety to the flavour of foods, herbs and spices are often rich in nutrients such as minerals. For instance, ginger contains iron, zinc and magnesium; fresh parsley is rich in carotene and vitamin C. Some women enjoy spicy foods more than usual in pregnancy but others find it is best to avoid them.

THREE

Does Weight Matter?

Whenever food is the subject of discussion, questions about weight and slimming almost invariably arise. Is being slim a good idea for pregnancy? Is it a good idea to go on a diet before you get pregnant in order to offset the weight gain later? Is it really necessary to carefully control how much weight you gain during pregnancy? If you gain quite a bit of weight during pregnancy, is it going to stay with you forever?

Emphasis has already been put on *what* you eat, but your ability to conceive, have a healthy baby and breast-feed well, is also dependent on *how much* you eat and what you weigh. It is not only the weight you gain during pregnancy which matters but also what you weigh before you even conceive. If you are still at the stage of planning a pregnancy, the following information will help you to work out a desirable weight for yourself. If you are already pregnant, taking your pre-pregnancy weight into account will help you to calculate what might be the best weight gain for you during pregnancy.

Your weight before pregnancy

Taking your weight into consideration, your height provides a general indication as to whether you are eating enough, too little or too much and whether you are taking enough exercise, too little or even possibly too much. The exceptions are caused by certain medical conditions which may affect the weight of a few individuals. In theory this sounds pretty straightforward but how much you eat might be affected by many things other than hunger, including stress, anxiety, depression, the time of the month, your vitamin and mineral status and last but by no means least, social stresses. Today's society has become so obsessed with weight and its control that messages intended for the very obese are even causing normal-weight individuals to make their lives miserable by slimming and trying to keep their weight below what is normal for them. Disorders like anorexia, binge-eating, compulsive eating and bulimia nervosa (compulsive eating followed by self-induced vomiting) are becoming increasingly common.

Some body fat is essential. In order to be able to menstruate normally and be able to conceive, most women need to have about twenty-five per cent of their weight as fat, and usually achieve this around the time of puberty. However, women who are very underweight – perhaps after an illness or due to dieting – may become temporarily infertile and unable to conceive until they gain some weight. Underweight women who do conceive naturally or under medical treatment have been found to be more likely to give birth to smaller babies than women of normal weight. At the other end of the scale, excessively overweight women may be slightly more at risk of menstrual irregularities and problems in pregnancy than average.

Since what a woman weighs is obviously related to her height, it has been recommended that women who are underweight or very overweight should be encouraged to achieve a more average weight for their height before they contemplate pregnancy. Inevitably this raises the vexed question of what is a desirable weight for height in pregnancy, or for that matter, for good health in general? Some of the much used charts based on frame size are now known to be of dubious merit. Equally unhelpful may be slimming advice in some magazines, where the term 'overweight' may indicate the smallest pinch of extra fat on waist or thighs and bear little or no relationship to health.

How can you know if you are the right weight for you?
Bathroom scales and calorie counters are useful on occasions and for certain individuals. Unfortunately, they have become almost objects of ritual. If you feel well, eat a well-balanced and nutritious diet of mostly unrefined foods, are physically active, do not get unduly exhausted by the rigours of daily existence and are not out of breath after climbing a flight of stairs, then it is quite likely that your weight is normal for you.

Does Weight Matter?

If, however, you are not content with this definition and hanker for technical precision, let Quetelet come to your rescue. He was a Belgian who, in the last century, weighed and measured large numbers of people and consequently came up with a useful guide to weight and height. This is now known as the Quetelet index and it is equal to your weight in kilograms divided by twice your height in metres i.e.

$$\text{Quetelet index} = \frac{\text{wt in kg}}{(\text{ht in m})^2}$$

This means, of course, that you have to measure your height in metres and your weight in kilograms or you can use the conversion table on page 40 to convert your weight in stones and pounds to kilograms and your height in feet and inches to metres. Then it is a simple matter to work out your index figure, and if this is between 20 and 25, you are in the desirable range for pregnancy. A little bit higher than 25 would not matter and is better than being below 20. An index of less than 20 puts you in the category of being underweight; an index of over 30 puts you in the very overweight classification.

Underweight – index less than 20

Janet, 5 ft 3 in (1.60 m) tall and weighing 7 st 8 lb (48.1 kg) had a Q index of 18.8. If your index is less than 20 and/or your periods are scanty, irregular or have ceased, you tire easily, have little enthusiasm for physical exertion, and conscientiously limit how much you eat, then it is likely that you are underweight. To gain weight you may need not only to eat more but to eat more often. Do not attempt enormous meals if your small stomach is unaccustomed to them. Instead eat three main meals with nutritious snacks in between. If you are not prepared to give up your skinny image for the sake of pregnancy, then it is worth considering which is more important to you, having a healthy baby or being sylph-like. For some women it is not possible to achieve both these aims – they have to make a conscious choice. If this is difficult because you feel you may be verging on anorexia, try to bring yourself to seek help from

Eating Well for a Healthy Pregnancy

Weight (st lb to kg   1 lb = 0.454 kg)

st	lb	kg	st	lb	kg	st	lb	kg
7	0	44.5	9	0	57.2	11	0	69.9
	1	44.9		1	57.6		1	70.3
	2	45.4		2	58.1		2	70.8
	3	45.8		3	58.5		3	71.2
	4	46.3		4	59.0		4	71.7
	5	46.7		5	59.4		5	72.1
	6	47.2		6	59.9		6	72.6
	7	47.6		7	60.3		7	73.0
	8	48.1		8	60.8		8	73.5
	9	48.5		9	61.2		9	73.9
	10	49.0		10	61.7		10	74.4
	11	49.4		11	62.1		11	74.8
	12	49.9		12	62.6		12	75.3
	13	50.4		13	63.1		13	75.8
8	0	50.8	10	0	63.5	12	0	76.2
	1	51.3		1	64.0		1	76.7
	2	51.7		2	64.4		2	77.1
	3	52.2		3	64.9		3	77.6
	4	52.6		4	65.3		4	78.1
	5	53.1		5	65.8		5	78.5
	6	53.5		6	66.2		6	79.0
	7	54.0		7	66.7		7	79.5
	8	54.4		8	67.1			
	9	54.9		9	67.6	13	0	82.6
	10	55.3		10	68.0			
	11	55.8		11	68.5	13	7	85.8
	12	56.3		12	69.0			
	13	56.7		13	69.4	14	0	89.0

Height (ft in to metres   1 in = 2.54 cm or 0.0254 m.   1 ft = 0.305 m)

ft	in	m	ft	in	m	ft	in	m
4	8	1.42	5	2	1.57	5	8	1.72
	9	1.45		3	1.60		9	1.75
	10	1.47		4	1.62		10	1.77
	11	1.50		5	1.65		11	1.80
5	0	1.52		6	1.67	6	0	1.83
	1	1.55		7	1.70		1	1.86

Example   5 ft 4 in = 162 cm or 1.62 m
9 st 3 lb = 58.5 kg

Quetelet index = $\dfrac{\text{wt in kg}}{(\text{ht in m})^2} = \dfrac{58.5}{1.62 \times 1.62} = 22.3$

Does Weight Matter?

your doctor and contact Anorexic Aid at the address given on page 147.

Deliberate food restriction may not be your particular problem; you may have tried eating more and still cannot gain weight. The first thing is to have a medical check up to make sure there is no medical reason for your low weight. If there is not, your doctor may suggest that you see a dietitian for specific advice on how to gain weight, and perhaps give the quality of your diet an overhaul too, since certain vitamin or mineral deficiencies might be affecting your appetite. Excessive anxiety or stress can also affect your weight, as too can extremes of physical activity.

If you are slim but light-boned, are menstruating normally, eat like the proverbial horse but choose a wide range of foods and feel well, then you may have no need to worry about your weight. However, do check that you are eating at least the number of portions recommended from the four food groups detailed in Chapter 2 – that you eat four to five items from the bread and cereals list; potatoes and carrots as well as green leaves from the vegetable group; a mixture of milk products and also at least two portions from the meat and alternatives group (more if you take tiny portions).

Quetelet index of 20-25

Sandra was 5 ft 4 in tall and weighed 9 st 3 lb. Her Quetelet index was 58.5 divided by 1.62 twice, that is, 22.3. If, like her, you have a Quetelet index between 20 and 25, then you will be among the majority. This is fine, both for your own health and for pregnancy. This range is not a sliding scale, which means that if your index is 25 or just below your health will not benefit in any way if you lose weight and make your index less. For you, weight is not a matter for concern; concentrate all your efforts on the quality of what you eat.

Quetelet index of 26-30

If your index is over 25, like Margaret who at 5 ft 2 in (1.57 m) weighed 10 st 10 lb (68 kg) and had a Quetelet index of 27.6, you are over average weight but only slightly so. The longterm risk to your health appears to be negligible. A couple of hundred years ago, women who were considered attractive and featured in paintings of the era, may have had an index of 26 or so. The only real danger of being in this range is that you may gain more weight and reach an index of more than 30.

Overweight – Quetelet index of more than 30
At 5 ft 6 in (1.67 m) tall, and 13 st 7 lb (85.8 kg), Jill had an index of 30.8. If you have an index over 30, like Jill, you are overweight and are more at risk than normal weight women of having problems with your own health and with pregnancy. During pregnancy you may be more likely to experience high blood pressure and to develop diabetes ('gestational' diabetes). Ideally, you should lose some weight well before you intend to start a baby and stabilize at this new weight for some time before you stop contraception.

How to lose weight: Losing weight is for some a seemingly insoluble problem. The book *Dieting Makes You Fat* by Geoffrey Cannon and Hetty Einsig (see reading list, page 143) gives many good reasons why diets so often fail, and how and why exercise and good food can help. If you are fat because you eat far too much, it may be that you overeat as a reaction to stress, loneliness or depression. Your need may be more for psychological help rather than a diet sheet. Perhaps, though, you do not eat a lot and may even eat less than your slimmer friends and workmates. In this case, it may be the wrong choice of foods and/or insufficient exercise over the course of several years which have contributed to your problem. Highly refined foods are often high calorie foods, and they do not fill you up like more wholesome foods so it is easy to eat more than you need. Some tactics you can try to help you lose some weight are given below:

1. Cut out all white bread, sugar, sweets, soft drinks, chocolate, cakes and biscuits.

2. Correct any possible deficiencies of vitamins and minerals by concentrating on a well-balanced diet from all four food groups, listed in Chapter 2. Do not overemphasize one type of food such as meat and neglect wholemeal bread,

Does Weight Matter?

potatoes, fruit and vegetables which should form a significant part of your diet. Lots of these fibre-rich foods will help you to feel full.

3. Eat three small but regular meals a day plus nutritious low calorie snacks. Missing meals almost inevitably leads to failure. One of the reasons for this is that people who starve themselves during the day and then eat in the evening, can often end up actually eating more than they might have done as small meals spaced throughout the day.

4. Increase your level of exercise – not by rushing off to a squash court or exercise class once a week but by your daily level of activity together with some form of exercise, two or three times a week, which makes you out of breath. The aim should be to increase the rate at which your body 'ticks over'. Get yourself moving every day in as brisk a way as possible – half-an-hour's brisk walk, using stairs rather than lifts whenever feasible. These and other tactics will help to speed up your body's functions and begin to burn up that extra fat. This will occur not only while you are exercising but will continue for some hours afterwards. You will begin to feel fitter and brighter. Next time you feel like eating and it is not a meal or snack time, get up and *do* something active.

5. Help your body to improve its ability to adapt to cold. Keeping your own body warm from within burns up units of heat (calories) and is economical! Be brave, turn down the central heating and throw out your bedwarmer.

If you are very overweight, do not be overambitious at first or you will be disappointed in your progress. Start slowly and steadily. Walking is an ideal beginning. The changes you make are for the longterm not just for the next few weeks or months. Resolutions to start a 'crash' diet tomorrow are often broken and depress you even more. Think positive. Concentrate on any progress you *have* achieved each week rather than on any failed targets or relapses.

Eventually this approach should work and you will settle into the weight category which is right for you. Your dilemma may be that you cannot wait for 'eventually' because you are approaching your mid-thirties or for some other reason

Eating Well for a Healthy Pregnancy

need to become pregnant soon. Discuss with your doctor the pros and cons of getting pregnant or of waiting until your weight is less. If you do become pregnant while very overweight, take great care to minimize all other risks (such as smoking and alcohol) and make sure you eat a sensible, balanced diet. A fat woman who is eating a well-balanced diet will be much healthier and more likely to have a normal pregnancy than the fat woman who eats lots of highly refined foods, sugar, biscuits, cakes and sweets and who may be malnourished in terms of vitamins and minerals. However overweight you may be, do *not* go on a strict low-calorie slimming diet during pregnancy (see next section).

Your weight during pregnancy

At the antenatal clinic, a common topic of conversation may be the 'weight' which has or has not been gained. Women come in all shapes and sizes and 'normal' weight gain during pregnancy can vary enormously. Yet often you are advised to gain between 24 and 28 lb during pregnancy, although healthy babies have been born to women who gained less than this and, indeed, to those who have gained more than twice the 2 st norm. If you eat to appetite of the foods already described, you should gain the amount appropriate for *you*, even if this differs from the average and from the weight gained in pregnancy by the girl next to you in the clinic, your friend, sister or neighbour. The weight that you gain is made up of all kinds of new tissues. In the case of a woman who gained 2 st during pregnancy and whose baby weighed 8 lb, the other 20 lb distributed in her body could be accounted for, in approximate terms, as follows:

weight of baby	8 lb	or	3.6 kg
placenta	1½ lb		0.7 kg
'waters'	1¾ lb		0.8 kg
increased breast size	1 lb		0.5 kg
increased size of womb	2½ lb		1.1 kg
extra fluid	5½ lb		2.5 kg
increase in fat store	7¾ lb		3.5 kg
	28 lb		12.7 kg

Does Weight Matter?

How is this weight put on during the course of pregnancy? Taking a weight gain of 28 lb as an example, some textbooks suggest that it might be put on in the following way:

extra weight at 10 weeks	1½ lb	or	0.7 kg
20 weeks	9 lb		4.1 kg
30 weeks	19 lb		8.6 kg
40 weeks	28 lb		12.7 kg

Do not expect yourself necessarily to conform to this textbook Mrs. Average. It can give you an approximate idea of how you may gain weight – but weight increase during pregnancy is a very individual matter. It may follow the above pattern or you may gain a similar total amount but at a different rate at each stage of pregnancy – or your pattern of weight gain may be completely different. Some women find that they are ravenous in early pregnancy and grow out of their normal clothes well before twelve weeks but then gain weight more slowly later on. Others may be so sick during the first three months that they actually lose weight, in which case they often go on to eat in order to regain lost ground and put on a lot of weight between twelve and thirty weeks.

If disturbing comments about weight are made at the antenatal clinic, because it is considered that you have gained too little or too much, what can you do? A common reaction is to keep quiet when the comments are made, then worry on returning home. This will not do you or the baby any good, so be brave – after all, the staff are there for the sole purpose of helping you to have as healthy a baby as possible. Discuss the issue openly and describe more fully the pattern of your weight gain (and possibly that of a previous pregnancy). If it becomes apparent that you are eating properly even though you do not fit the text book ideal, then your weight 'problem' might resolve itself. In any case, at least you should get further advice and clarification.

If you do not gain much after thirty weeks, and you are eating well, do not be alarmed. Talk it over at the antenatal clinic. Just make sure you are still eating *enough* – this may mean taking small frequent meals rather than attempting three large meals a day. Do *not* eat less during these last crucial weeks. You can assess how well the baby is doing by the movements he or she makes when awake. These movements may slacken off just before labour but if the movements become less frequent than usual *before* this time, let your doctor or midwife know.

What you can do if underweight during pregnancy
Jane was 5 ft 4 in tall (1.62 m) and weighed 7 st 13 lb (50.4 kg) before pregnancy. She felt and ate well during pregnancy and gained more than the average amount of weight. In fact, the 36 lb she gained could be accounted for by 28 lb for pregnancy and an 8 lb gain to bring her own non-pregnant weight up to 8 st 7 lb (54.0 kg) which would give her a Q index of 20.6.

If your actual weight before conception gave you an index below 20, you too may need to put on more than average weight in pregnancy to allow for this. At the antenatal clinic be sure to say how much you weighed before pregnancy and that you were perhaps underweight. Do *not* limit what you eat during pregnancy to try and keep your weight gain low, or you may be at risk of having a smaller than average baby.

What you can do if overweight during pregnancy
Do *not* go on a strict diet; eat to appetite. However, this should not be taken as a licence to indulge in low quality, high-calorie foods. Select nutritious and mostly unrefined foods from the four food groups listed in Chapter 2 and you will automatically exclude the highly processed and high-calorie foods with a low value for health. Your weight gain may then turn out to be that which is best for you personally. This may be less than the 28 lb average – you may gain weight for all the items listed at the beginning of this section, except for the $7\frac{3}{4}$ lb fat store, since your fat store is already ample enough. A low calorie diet is not advisable because there seems to be no beneficial effect either to mother or baby. Even well-supervised efforts to restrict women's diets during pregnancy have not always produced the desired effect. Some overweight women who dieted after the thirtieth week of pregnancy did gain a few pounds less than non-dieters but most of this saved weight

Does Weight Matter?

was fluid. Less than 1 lb was due to fat, hardly a significant saving. Nor was it beneficial that they gained less fluid, despite the belief by some that this would lessen the risk of pre-eclampsia, a potentially dangerous medical condition of pregnancy (see page 106). Strict low calorie diets do not lessen this risk, indeed it is the opinion of some people that they may increase it in pregnancy.

If you are overweight you may need to take particular care over what you eat in the last few months – care to eat properly. It is quite likely that after the thirtieth week you will be less interested in food, since your stomach will be squashed by the baby and by your own abdominal fat. Meanwhile, your baby is growing fast and although he or she can take some advantage of your fat stores, it will not be possible to survive on them entirely. It may be difficult to imagine starvation in the midst of plenty, but this could happen. The baby needs an input of protein and carbohydrate and could be choked by the fat and other substances which are produced if you live almost entirely off your own reserves. So eat enough frequent small meals made up from the four food groups to keep your system working well. Postpone any intentions about losing weight until after the birth, but completely cut out sweets, chocolate, cakes, biscuits and high calorie drinks.

Your weight after the birth

Nothing can compare with the joy of holding your baby for the first time, nor with that wonderful feeling of having shed such an enormous burden of weight. You feel positively light-footed and so slim. It may be with a sense of delight or perhaps trepidation that you first approach a pair of scales after the birth; or you may decide to ignore them altogether.

What should you expect to weigh after the birth? It is generally considered average for a woman to be about 9 lb (4.1 kg) above the weight she was before pregnancy. Most women, especially those who breast-feed, lose this weight within a few months after delivery. But in some cases the extra weight may be lost more slowly, or occasionally not at all. The finding that some women tend to get heavier with

Eating Well for a Healthy Pregnancy

each successive pregnancy is usually related more to increasing age and reduced physical activity than to pregnancy itself.

What you can do if underweight after the birth
Once you are back at home and busy looking after the baby, it may not be easy to get your weight back up to normal. If you are underweight you may tire more easily and perhaps be put off breast-feeding. ('But you're far too small dear to feed *him* – he's such a big baby.') Although you may not have the accumulated fat stores to aid lactation that the average woman may have, there is still no reason why you should not breast-feed successfully. It just means that you need to eat sufficient for your own daily needs plus some for regaining lost weight and extra still for feeding the baby. Do not embark on any violent exercise programme yet and try to avoid emotional stress, both of which could spell disaster to your chances of gaining weight and of breast-feeding.

What you can do if overweight after the birth
It is completely irrational to expect to be back to your normal weight in a matter of weeks, let alone days, but you may still feel rather depressed when all your attempts to tuck yourself into your old clothes fail and you put on that maternity dress yet again.

If this *is* your experience, try to see your weight change over an eighteen-month rather than a nine-month period. It took nine months to put on and it may take nine months to get back to normal. Nature intended that to continue to provide for your baby, you should store extra weight on your abdomen, hips, thighs and breasts. Breast-feeding really will help you to get your figure back but do not cut back on your rations. Your baby is still just as dependent on you as when in the womb. See yourself not as overweight but as breastfeeding weight. To cheer yourself up treat yourself to an attractive new outfit with easy front openings above the waist.

Even after months of breast-feeding some women stubbornly remain a good half a stone heavier, often around the breasts, upper arms, abdomen and hips.

Does Weight Matter?

Sometimes it is only after breast-feeding stops that the surplus weight is lost. Within a few weeks of finally weaning the baby, your weight will probably go back to normal. If this is not the case and you still remain overweight, follow the strategies already outlined for pre-pregnancy overweight problems. As the baby gets older you will begin to take more exercise yourself and if you do not eat any more, then you will slowly lose the excess weight. Check too, from the Quetelet index (see page 40), that you really do have a weight problem in terms of health rather than one which is solely related to fashion.

FOUR

Putting Theory Into Practice

Feeling confident about your weight and knowing which foods to eat for a healthy diet represent only the first stage of good nutrition for pregnancy; the quality of the food you buy, the way that you store, prepare and cook it may all have a marked impact on the nutritional value of what you finally eat. Food which is chosen well, stored well and prepared well, will be better food for both you and the baby. Good habits developed before and during pregnancy will set a trend too for healthy food for your child when he or she is growing up.

Shopping for food

Unless you have your own transport, shopping can be difficult when you are pregnant, especially if you already have one or more infants to take with you everywhere. Early and late pregnancy are usually the most tiring times so limit your weekday shopping to basic essentials and try to recruit some help with the heavier items in a once-a-week stocking-up session.

Also, plan ahead for the first hectic weeks after the baby is born. Write out a week's or fortnight's simple eating plan and make a shopping list so that it is one thing less to think about at that time. If finances permit, stock up on basic items which will store for a few weeks without deteriorating – dried fruit, nuts, pulses, brown rice, pasta, frozen foods, and canned foods such as sardines or other fish, Italian tomatoes and pineapple or other fruit in its own juice. If you own a freezer, put away some made-up dishes.

When pregnancy is advanced, ambitious economy trips involving long bus or train journeys may not be worth the extra time and effort involved. If you must go on such an outing, take a snack with you. Find somewhere to sit down so you can have ten minutes rest; if necessary ask for a chair

Putting Theory Into Practice

but don't wait until you get to the stage of feeling faint.

With such an enormous choice of foods available, shopping is a strategic exercise – balancing finances, satisfying preferences, assessing which foods are nutritious and good value, and reading labels to find out what additives are present.

For small specialist shops such as a butcher, fishmonger, grocer or greengrocer, choose one which attracts lots of custom. You may have to queue sometimes but value for money is likely to be good and the quick food turnover will ensure fresh produce.

In a supermarket you are up against the clever marketing expertise of wealthy multi-national companies, whose interest is in persuading you to spend money. Foods with a high profit margin but not necessarily good for health may be temptingly displayed in eye-catching places, whilst less expensive but nutritive basics are usually at the back of the store. Have a clear idea of what you need beforehand – it's a good idea to make a list – and go straight to the shelves you want. Become a label reader (see the booklet *Look at the Label*, mentioned in the reading list on page 144). By law, most prepared and processed foods must list all the ingredients in descending order by weight. Choose foods that are as simple and as unadulterated as possible, and this will help to exclude foods which are highly refined and processed or which contain a lot of artificial colourings, preservatives and additives. Fruit and vegetables can be expensive in supermarkets but they are usually very fresh and of good quality.

It is true that food costs a lot, but a good healthy diet need cost no more than the 'average' diet. Two shoppers can go into the same supermarket and spend exactly the same amount of money, yet come out with quite different baskets in terms of nutritional value. In the table on pages 52 and 53 are listed two weekly shopping baskets such as may be bought for a family of four. The contents of these baskets were identical in total cost and purchased in the same supermarket, but there the similarities end.

From basket A, you could prepare main meal menus such as roast chicken with jacket potatoes and sprouts followed by yogurt; or lamb's liver with onions and mashed potatoes,

Eating Well for a Healthy Pregnancy

Contents of two shopping baskets, equal in price, purchased in the same supermarket

BASKET A

Meat and alternatives

1 lb beef mince
1 chicken
¾ lb lamb's liver
4 pork chops
1 rabbit
2 tins of sardines
1 lb fish
2 doz eggs
2 tins of baked beans
½ lb hazelnuts

Bread and cereals

5 large wholemeal loaves
1 kg rolled oats
2 packets of rye crispbread
½ lb rice
1.5 kg wholemeal flour
4 oz wheatgerm
500 g macaroni

Milk and milk products

28 pints of milk
1 lb cheese
large natural yogurt
3 packets of butter

Vegetables and fruit

10 lb potatoes
2 tins of tomatoes
1 lb beetroot
3 lb cabbage
3 lb carrots
2 lb onions
1 lb sprouts
2 lb cauliflower
1 lettuce
½ lb tomatoes
bunch of watercress
½ cucumber
2 lb bananas
6 lb oranges
2 lb apples
2 lb grapefruit
4 peaches
2 lb pears
packet of stoned dates
packet of sultanas
2 cartons of orange juice

Miscellaneous

1 oz yeast
1 jar of honey

BASKET B

Meat and alternatives

1 large tin of steak
Tandoori cooked chicken
2 tins of luncheon meat
4 pork pies
8 beefburgers
2 jars of fish paste
10 fishfingers
2 jars of frankfurters
1 lb pork sausage
4 sausage rolls

Bread and cereals

5 large white loaves
large packet of sugar puffs
large packet of cornflakes
2 tins of rice pudding
3 pizzas
2 packets of cream crackers
2 packets of semi-sweet biscuits
2 packets of sandwich biscuits
2 tins of macaroni cheese

Putting Theory Into Practice

Vegetables and fruit

4 lb frozen oven chips
large instant mash
2 tins of processed peas
2 large tins of carrots
1 packet of dried vegetable soup
1 packet of instant tomato soup
12 packets of crisps
2 jars of jam
1 jar of marmalade
6 jam tarts
1 large tin of fruit salad
1 large tin of peaches

Milk and milk products

7 pints skimmed milk
1 tin of dried milk
½ lb processed cheese
½ lb cheese spread
4 cheesecakes

Miscellaneous

3 packets of margarine
1 packet of jelly
1 litre non-dairy ice-cream
1 packet of sugar
1 packet of sweets
1 litre 'orange' drink
6 bars of chocolate
2 litres cola drink

with peaches for 'afters'. Lunch or supper dishes could include vegetable and chicken soup (using the carcass from the roast chicken) with wholemeal bread; cheese, tomato and onion pizza (using the wholemeal flour and yeast); sardine salad; or macaroni cheese. Not only can you prepare your own macaroni cheese and pizza, but have enough money left for salad and fresh fruit to serve alongside. Snacks from basket A might include nuts and sultanas, fruit, bread and honey, with fruit juice or milk to drink.

In comparison, the menus which can be put together from basket B are not so well-balanced and the snacks, biscuits, sweets, and chocolate bars and the soft drinks are rich in calories but poor in nutritional value.

The chart on page 54 illustrates the relative proportions of nutrients in basket B compared with basket A. As you can see, basket B contains a greater proportion of calories, fat and sugar which we are often recommended to cut back on. We are also advised to eat more unsaturated fat and fibre, which are better represented in basket A. In fact, basket A contains twice as many of the essential polyunsaturated fatty acids, linoleic and linolenic, as basket B. The table also shows that basket B contains a much lower proportion of vitamins such as vitamin A, C and folate and of minerals such as zinc, copper and magnesium. Finally, basket B contains many more non-food items – colourings,

Eating Well for a Healthy Pregnancy

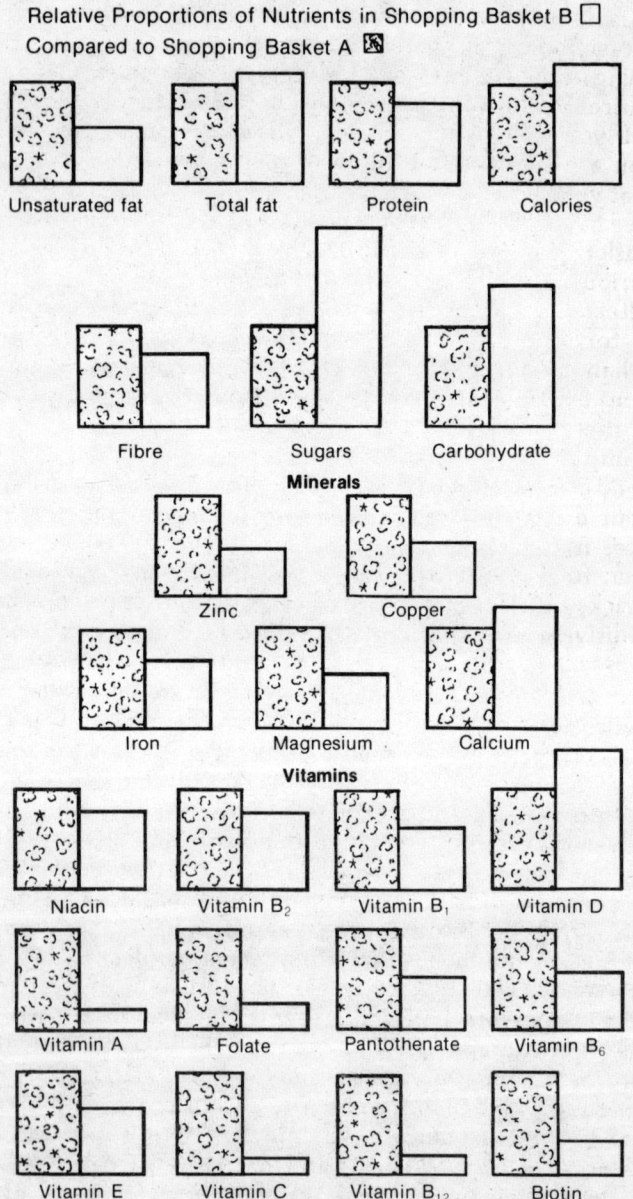

preservatives, and other additives – than basket A. The occasional use of highly refined and processed foods is not going to be harmful but total reliance on a diet made up entirely of such foods will eventually take its toll on health.

If you have to manage on a very low income, check that you are receiving all the income/supplements/allowances that you should be getting, and whether you are entitled to free milk while you are pregnant. Ask at your local clinic for leaflet FB8 'Babies and Benefits' which describes all the various benefits and how to find out more about them. Alternatively write for this leaflet to the DHSS leaflet unit or for other information about benefits to the Maternity Alliance or the National Council for One-parent Families (see p. 149). It may be necessary to economize on clothes, furnishings, even light and heating, but never skimp on food. Your baby won't complain about second-hand clothes or passed-on cot but both of you may suffer if your diet is inadequate. However, not skimping on food does not mean that you cannot economize. Prepare your own food and it will always be cheaper than readymade snacks and meals, and you will avoid paying for non-food additives, colourings and packagings. If you can afford a pressure cooker, this can be very cost-saving on fuel.

A low cost diet for pregnancy which would be adequate in the major nutrients, protein, fat and carbohydrate and the vitamins and minerals is shown in the table on page 56. You can economize by buying cheaper, but not necessarily less nutritive, cuts of meat – and offal is excellent value; buy coley not haddock, herring not tuna; brown bananas and baked beans. Use fish heads for stocks and soups, bones for stock, older cheese to make sandwich spread or cheese pudding (poor man's soufflé), day-old wholemeal bread for toast, and why not make your own yogurt? Supplement the protein in small portions of meat and sausage with cereals (pastry or pasta) or with pulses served in a casserole together with vegetables.

Basic low cost diet

Shopping list At 1984 prices, this diet worked out at approximately £1.60 a day. (Continued overleaf.)

Eating Well for a Healthy Pregnancy

Meat and alternatives

Stewing steak	3 oz
Mince	3 oz
Pork chop (meat)	3 oz
Haddock	8 oz
Lamb's liver	4 oz
Pork sausage	3 oz
7 eggs	420 g
Baked beans	450 g
Tin of sardines	120 g
Fresh peanuts	2 oz
Frozen peas	250 g
Butter beans (dried)	100 g

Bread and cereals

Porridge oats	350 g
Wholemeal bread	1 kg
Wholemeal flour	4 oz
Rice (uncooked)	50 g
Digestive biscuits	250 g

Vegetables and fruit

Old potatoes	5 lb
Cabbage	1¾ lb
Carrots	2¼ lb
Brussels sprouts	½ lb
Box of mustard and cress	25 g
Bananas	1 lb
7 oranges	2 lb
Apples	2 lb
Chopped dates	4 oz
Onions	1 lb
Tin of tomatoes	400 g

Milk and milk products

Milk	7 pints
Cheese	8 oz
Butter	150 g
Natural yogurt (to make own yogurt)	150 g

Miscellaneous

Yeast extract	56 g
Lard	50 g
Sugar	100 g
Packet of tea	125 g

Nutrients supplied

Calories	2400
Protein	103 g
Vitamin A	3488 µg**
Carotene	16 608 µg
Vitamin D	2.8 µg*
Vitamin E	6.9 mg
Vitamin B_1	2.1 mg
Vitamin B_2	3.8 mg
Niacin	24 mg
Vitamin B_6	2.3 mg
Vitamin B_{12}	18 µg
Pantothenate	8.0 mg
Folate	478 µg
Biotin	57 µg
Vitamin C	135 mg
Calcium	1480 mg
Magnesium	516 mg
Iron	18 mg
Zinc	16 mg
Copper	3.5 mg

* extra comes from sunlight
** exceeds the RDA but excess vitamin A from food is not a problem as the body adjusts and absorbs less carotene.

An example of an economy diet is given here. In the shopping list above, the amounts given are those used for the purposes of calculating what this example of a diet supplies in terms of

Putting Theory Into Practice

calories, protein, vitamins and minerals. They may not be exactly those which you would buy as you may be shopping for more than one person. Also one particular purchase e.g. flour, oats, rice, may contain much more than the amount given. The next week, however, this item would not need to be bought.

Basic low cost diet

Weekly menu
Below are some simple suggestions for meals, from the shopping basket above, but other alternatives are possible.

☐ *Breakfasts*
   1 orange; home-made muesli (oats, fruit, dates, nuts) or porridge; boiled egg; (except Sunday, no egg).
   1 slice wholemeal toast and butter.

☐ *Milk*
   1 pint a day (in drinks, on cereal, by itself, in yogurt and rice pudding).

☐ *Snacks*
   Digestive biscuits, nuts, dates, fruit, bread, yogurt.

☐ *Drinks*
   milk, tea, yeast extract.

☐ *Sunday*
   lunch: Stewing steak, peas, Brussels sprouts, roast potatoes, apple pie and cheese (1 oz).
   supper: Vegetable soup (e.g. carrots, onions, cabbage, peas, potatoes), poached egg and 2 slices wholemeal bread.

☐ *Monday*
   lunch: 2 slices wholemeal bread and sardines. Winter salad (cabbage, carrots, onion, dates), 1 banana.
   supper: Butter bean, tomato and onion casserole with cheese (½ oz) topping. Cabbage and mashed potatoes. Remainder of apple pie and yogurt.

☐ *Tuesday*
   lunch: 2 slices wholemeal bread and 2 oz cheese, mustard & cress, raw carrot, apple.
   supper: Pork chop, Brussels sprouts, jacket potatoes, butter beans (cooked for Monday supper), rice pudding.

☐ *Wednesday*
   lunch: 2 slices wholemeal bread and sardines (stored in icebox section of fridge). Winter salad (cabbage, carrot, apple).
   supper: Lamb's liver and onions, carrots and potatoes, biscuits and cheese (½ oz).

☐ *Thursday*
   lunch: 2 slices wholemeal bread and 2 oz cheese. Cress and raw carrot. Apple.
   supper: Mince, peas, cabbage, potatoes, banana and yogurt (made on Monday from yogurt plus milk, and kept in fridge).

☐ *Friday*
   lunch: 2 slices wholemeal bread and baked beans. Salad (carrot, cheese, cress), apple.
   supper: Haddock, peas and chips. Biscuits and cheese (1 oz).

☐ *Saturday*
   lunch: Cheese rarebit (1 oz cheese) and baked beans. Apple.
   supper: Pork sausage, cabbage, baked potato, rice pudding and banana.

Experience will tell you that economizing on food need not jeopardize your nutritional status – and if you look upon it as an interesting challenge, you can get a lot of satisfaction out of devising new and nourishing menus. However, experience makes you realize that at times you weary of scrounging and scraping, so hopefully you may even save enough to justify splashing out every now and again on a special treat.

Storage of food

Manufacturers and food processors are often criticized for what they do to food but we should also be critical of our own methods of food storage and preparation since we, too, can greatly affect the nutritional value of what we eat.

The old maxim 'Eat only those foods which readily rot, go stale or go sour but eat them *before* they do so' is still relevant today. Fresh and wholesome foods, rich in nutrients, are also attractive to bacteria and moulds and deteriorate easily. The enemies of many foods are warmth, light and moisture, because micro-organisms thrive in these conditions, because rancidity of fats can occur and because unstable vitamins can be damaged.

Cool, dark and dry storage conditions pose no problems if you live in an old house with basement, cellar or cool larder, but proper storage can be a headache if you have a new, central-heated house or flat with a tiny kitchen and no shed or garage. Here the only solution is to refrigerate what you

Putting Theory Into Practice

can and buy dry goods (cereals, bread, flour and dried fruit and nuts) in small quantities as you need them. If you have some spare space and money, it may be worth investing in a second (and secondhand?) fridge, in which to keep fruit and vegetables.

Storing meat and alternatives

Remove any plastic wrapping on fresh meat, poultry and fish on return home, put the food in a covered dish and refrigerate. The more finely cut up meat is, the quicker it will spoil, so use mince more quickly than a joint. Use sausages quickly, too, especially if you have asked your butcher to make them without artificial preservatives and colour. If you buy frozen poultry, allow plenty of time for it to thaw right through before cooking. Poultry trimmings or giblets spoil quickly and should be cooked for stock or sauce as soon as possible. After removing the meat from cooked poultry, cover the carcass with water, add a bayleaf and simmer to make stock – use in soup, gravy or sauce or freeze in half-pint cartons for use within the next few months (small cartons thaw out more quickly than large).

The more fish smells, the older it is, so choose firm fish without a strong fishy odour. Look for bright eyes and scales in whole fish. Cook and eat fish, especially the very nutritious roe, on the day you buy it or, at the very latest, the next day.

Fresh eggs, when cracked open, have a high standing yolk and a white which clings to the yolk and sometimes to the shell. Older eggs have a flatter yolk and white which spreads out more. Use these up quickly. Otherwise store eggs in a cool airy place, not in the fridge, because they can absorb flavours very easily from other foods. Refrigerate cooked egg dishes and eat by the next day.

Dried peas, beans and lentils can be stored readily on an open shelf or in a cupboard but if you store them for months on end, they can become so hard that it is just about impossible to cook them tender. So if you use them only occasionally, buy in small amounts. The same applies to nuts. Chopped, flaked or ground nuts deteriorate even more quickly so buy only very tiny quantities as needed. Better still, invest in a small inexpensive nut mill to grind

Eating Well for a Healthy Pregnancy

whole nuts (which can work out cheaper) for use in muesli, baking, desserts etc. as needed.

Storing bread and cereals

Keep wholemeal bread cool (in an earthenware crock or wrapped in a teatowel). Extra loaves can be wrapped in greaseproof, then in a plastic bag and stored in the fridge for a few days, or in the freezer for a few weeks. Ten to fifteen minutes in a low oven will refresh bread, or pop rolls under a low grill if you like them crisp outside and soft inside. Older bread can be toasted, used for home-made breadcrumbs or for bread-and-butter or summer puddings.

Rice, cereals and pasta should also be kept cool, dark and dry (in opaque, airtight containers if you have them). Do not store very large quantities of flour, rolled oats, oatmeal etc., because once a grain is milled or rolled, some of the substances thus exposed to the air begin to spoil very quickly. Keep any surplus wholemeal flour sealed in a plastic bag in the fridge or for longer periods in the freezer.

Always keep wheatgerm in a tightly sealed bag in the fridge, especially untreated wheatgerm. This should be used within a few weeks so check its age when you buy. 'Stabilized' wheatgerm keeps longer, although it is slightly more processed.

Storing vegetables and fruit

Unpack any plastic-wrapped fruit and vegetables. Bananas hate the cold and should never be refrigerated, but most other fruits are best kept cool. Ideally, have a small selection of fresh fruit in a bowl at room temperature as they will taste better than if eaten from the cold, but keep the remainder in a cool place. Potatoes should be kept in the dark as well as cool or they will turn green, and the green parts are poisonous. Store salad vegetables in the fridge drawer; stand cut ends of lettuce and celery in a small amount of water in a cool place. Cover watercress completely with water – leaves as well as stalks – (it is grown in running water) but change the water frequently. Carrots and onions usually store quite well but leafy vegetables such as spinach, broccoli, spring cabbage soon wilt and lose value, so use within a short time.

Storing milk and milk products

Refrigerate milk as soon as possible after delivery; if it has to stand outside for any length of time, leave an insulated box in a shady spot, and ask your milkman to place the milk in it. This will also keep out the light, which can destroy one of the B vitamins, riboflavin or B_2.

A cool larder or cellar provides ideal conditions for storing cheese; if you cannot do this, well wrap the cut cheese surfaces but not the crust in clingfilm or foil before storing it in the nearest place to a cellar you can devise. If your fridge temperature is below 40°F, then it is really too cold for cheese. In warm weather buy only small quantities of cheese at a time or it may sweat excessively and become very strong-flavoured.

The preparation of food

Preparing meat and alternatives

Do not salt meat or fish before cooking because it draws out the natural juices. Treat the protein in all meat, fish and eggs with respect, by cooking for longer at moderate temperatures rather than for a short time at a very high temperature. Baste roast meat often with its own fat or add a little extra fat just for basting as this protects the meat from direct heat. Liver is a delicate meat – do not soak, wash or beat it but wipe carefully and sauté gently in a little butter or oil, or cook it in a casserole. If you eat liver because it is good for you rather than because you enjoy it, try some recipes which present it in different ways (see reading list on page 143). Prepare your own hamburgers from mince unless you know what is in the readymade ones.

Protect fish from intense temperatures by poaching, steaming, or baking wrapped in foil (with butter and herbs if you wish). Any water, milk or stock should just barely cover the fish. Grilling of fish is best reserved for fish steaks or small whole fish such as herring, mackerel or plaice; protect by brushing with melted butter or oil. Alternatively, dip in milk or egg first, roll lightly in flour, home-made breadcrumbs (commercial ones contain dye), bran, oats or fine oatmeal and fry gently.

Simmer rather than fast-boil eggs, fry or scramble

gently. When making egg custard, stand the pan of custard in or over a larger pan of simmering water (or use a double-boiler if you have one). A teaspoon of cornflour added at the mixing stage will help to stop custard curdling.

Many nutritious dishes are based on beans, peas or lentils. If you have not eaten them before, lentil soup or lentils in a stew are easy ones to try first, since lentils cook quickly. Most other pulses need long soaking (overnight) in cold water or, if you forget, an hour's soak in hot water (boil them for 2–3 minutes first). This is a preliminary to the cooking process, and after the soaking it is important to rinse the pulses thoroughly under the tap. Whatever method of cooking you use, you should boil them for at least ten minutes – this is to ensure that you destroy certain harmful substances present in the raw beans. Then they can be simmered gently until tender or cooked in a slow cooker for a long time. Beans can be cooked in a pressure cooker to economize on fuel and cooking time. More and more magazines now carry recipes for dishes based on pulses and *The Bean Book* by Rose Elliot (see p. 143) not only has lots of recipes and menu ideas but is a mine of information about the various pulses.

Preparing bread and cereals
Good quality wholemeal bread is now widely available but some women like to make their own. You may have tried and felt a failure because the loaf was miserably small and dense. This does not matter as long as you like the taste and do not object to the close texture. After all, the shop loaf only has extra air in it, made possible because commercial bakers have at their disposal all manner of techniques, special raising ovens and extra additives besides yeast, which all help to produce a larger, fluffier loaf.

How well home-made bread rises will also depend on the type of flour used. Flour from 'hard' wheat (usually North American) contains more gluten which makes bread rise more than flour from 'soft' wheat (most English wheat and organically grown wheat is 'soft'). Bread made from soft wheat flour tastes good but will not rise as much as bread from a hard gluten-rich flour. If you are still dissatisfied with your own bread, try using a slightly different method,

Putting Theory Into Practice

a different amount of liquid, a different brand of flour or a different recipe. Beginners can try buying a bread-making kit first. Follow the instructions closely until you've mastered techniques such as the kneading and right cooking temperature and then go on to buy all the ingredients separately.

Wholemeal flour can be very rough, so for other home baking (or for baby's first bread), either buy wheatmeal flour or sieve out the coarsest bran from wholemeal, or just use a proportion of wholemeal flour mixed with white in your usual pastry or cake recipes. This is one way, too, to introduce wholemeal bread to your family, increasing the amount of wholemeal flour gradually as they become accustomed to its taste and texture.

If the texture of muesli seems rather coarse at first, try soaking it overnight in milk. Add any fresh fruit just before eating. Creamy porridge can be made by soaking rolled oats or oatmeal in water overnight and cooking gently in the morning. Afterwards the stickiest porridge pan will become easy to clean if you just leave it full of cold water for a few hours. Another way to cook porridge is to put oatmeal and almost boiling water in a wide necked vacuum flask. Seal and leave overnight.

Brown rice and pasta take longer to cook than white. Rice should be cooked gently in a limited amount of simmering water in a lidded pan and stirred only once when it begins to simmer. If you disturb it more than this, the starch grains will burst and make the rice sticky. Pasta, in contrast, should be cooked vigorously in plenty of boiling water and kept on the move – also to prevent sticking. For rice as well as bean salads, add salad dressing to cooked rice or beans whilst still hot but after draining well. Then stir carefully and leave to cool. Add other salad ingredients just before serving.

Preparing vegetables and fruit

It is easy to say 'don't peel' or 'eat the whole fruit or vegetable', but this can conjure up thoughts of apple cores, banana skins and orange peel. Even monkeys peel their fruit. But don't peel unless necessary. Scrub vegetables clean and scrape or peel off any diseased parts, and be especially careful to cut out the poisonous green parts of potatoes. Baked potatoes in their jackets or new ones boiled in their skins are simple, taste good and conserve nutrients. If you prefer soft-skinned jacket potatoes, rub them with olive or other oil before baking. For quicker cooking, wrap each potato in foil or impale on a skewer or special potato rack (this will soon pay for itself in saved fuel).

Do not soak fresh vegetables in water for any length of time or vitamins and minerals will be lost. Cook them in as little water and for as short a time as possible – just until they are in-between crisp and tender. Diced cabbage may need only 5–10 minutes and spring or shredded cabbage even less.

Once vegetables are cut up finely, vitamins begin to be lost so, if possible, leave preparation until just before cooking and serving. Frozen vegetables can be cooked straight from frozen, need very little or no water and take less time to cook than fresh vegetables. Steaming of vegetables takes a little longer than boiling (try a colander over a pan of boiling water before investing in a collapsible steamer to fit different-sized pans). Another way to cook vegetables is stir-frying in oil. Traditionally a wok, a Chinese cooking vessel rather like a large, bowl-shaped frying pan, is used but a good quality large frying pan will serve the purpose. Cut up vegetables small and evenly and add them to the hot oil in sequence – those needing most cooking go in first.

Try different ways of serving vegetables. Beetroot cooked in its skin until tender then easily peeled is good served plain but raw young beetroot grated is equally delicious in a salad, as too is beetroot soup or beetroot cubed, cooked and served as a hot vegetable. 'Greens' can be used in a variety of ways besides as a main vegetable or salad (for example, chopped finely in a sandwich, quiche, cheese sauce or soup).

Homemade soup is entirely different from packet or tinned soup. It can make a nutritious start to a meal, is an extra way to serve vegetables, and can use up surplus gravy, stock, vegetable water and cooked leftovers. If meat, rice, barley or beans are added, it can be a meal in itself. Making soup is an art rather than an exact science, so you

Putting Theory Into Practice

can use your own imagination and what is at hand, but follow these basic rules as applicable:

1. Cut up hard vegetables finely and into evenly sized pieces so they cook evenly.

2. Sauté vegetables gently in butter, oil or dripping in a covered pan until soft but not brown (potatoes are sometimes added late in this process as they can stick).

3. Add stock, gravy and other ingredients (tomatoes, meat scraps, cooked beans, peas, rice etc) and simmer all until soft (approximately twenty minutes). Add any leftover cooked vegetables towards the end of simmering.

4. Serve the mixture up either as a rough broth or put it through a mouli-legume (a worthwhile investment – buy the largest you can afford, for fruit purées as well as soup). Alternatively, use a blender.

5. Further thickening or enrichment, if necessary, can come from milk, flour and milk (when the soup must be brought to the boil again to expand the starch granules in the flour) or, for special occasions, an egg liaison or cream (do not boil soup again when these are added).

Prepare salad vegetables and raw fruit dishes at the last minute before a meal. Dry vegetables carefully and well; do not bruise the more delicate ones such as lettuce. For the best results, toss vegetables in oil first to coat and protect the leaves, then add wine vinegar and any seasonings and toss again.

When making up a fresh fruit salad, dip slices of fruits which quickly discolour (apple, pear, banana) into a small bowl of lemon juice and water (or water and a pinch of citric acid – obtainable from most chemists). A useful base for a fruit salad is a tin of unsweetened pineapple to which a mixture of fresh fruit and/or soaked dried fruit is added.

If fresh fruit is to be cooked, do this gently in a little water, apple juice or other fruit juice, and poach until just tender (approximately 5 minutes on top of the cooker will suffice for gooseberries and blackberries but longer for whole apples, pears etc and longer, too, if cooked gently in the oven). If fruit discolours during cooking, next time try adding a pinch of vitamin C powder (obtainable from chemists) or a little lemon juice before cooking, and baste the fruit with this. Acid fruits can begin to dissolve the aluminium from aluminium pans so do not leave fruit in such pans after cooking or, better still, use non-aluminium pans for cooking acid fruits.

Planning ahead is needed for dried fruit (put to soak the night before or early in the morning for an evening meal) but it is well worth the little effort involved. Dried fruit may seem expensive, but a small amount swells a great deal in water. Dried fruit offer a great variety of dessert possibilities – puréed as a compôte with yogurt, cream or ice-cream, or left whole in a fruit salad or flan.

Preparing milk products

If you like yogurt, making your own is very economical and elaborate equipment is not necessary. Unless you are using milk straight from the cow or goat, you need to scald the milk first to kill any germs which might otherwise compete with the yogurt-making bacteria. Some people use special yogurt 'starter' culture but a small pot of ordinary unsweetened natural yogurt usually works well enough. Some yogurts are pasteurized so if one brand does not work well, try another make or some 'live' yogurt:

1. Scald 1–2 pints of milk by heating almost to boiling point and then leave to cool until skin temperature.
2. Stir in a few teaspoonsful of yogurt, cover and leave in a warm but not hot place in an opaque jug or container (for example on an Aga, in an airing cupboard or near a boiler, or in a vacuum flask).

2. *An alternative* is to place the yogurt mixture in small containers in a large lidded container with some warm water around the pots and at intervals replace the warm water.

3. Leave till thick; this takes about 12 hours but can vary from a few hours to a day or more. The longer it incubates, the stronger and more tart will be the yogurt.

4. When ready, keep in fridge until needed. Thicken and sweeten with fruit, fruit purée, honey etc.

Delicious ice-cream is also simple to make at home. It is

good enough for a special occasion now that real ice-cream is almost impossible to find or extremely expensive. Do not be deterred by lack of an ice-cream maker, which might give a creamier texture but is not essential. A good recipe to try first is one which uses a mixture of lightly whipped cream and a cooled home-made egg custard. Freeze in a shallow metal dish and, if you can remember, stir every twenty minutes to break up the ice crystals. Since this ice-cream is rather hard, take it out of the freezer and put it in the fridge for about half to one hour before serving so that it can soften. Mousses (and water ices made with fresh fruits) are also often appreciated more than highly complicated but over-rich desserts.

Cottage and cream cheese and even hard cheese can be made at home but, unlike yogurt, are not worth considering unless you keep a goat or cow or can obtain surplus milk very cheaply. Old or dried out cheese can be used for rarebit, 'buck' rarebit (rarebit topped with poached egg), a tomato-cheese sandwich spread or cheese pudding.

Eating patterns

When you are pregnant, don't make your baby wait long periods between meals. It does not make much biological sense to expect your body to run on stored nutrients for most of the day and then when it's tired, suddenly burden it with a large meal to digest. It makes even less sense when you are pregnant. So get into the habit of having breakfast. This is easy enough for early-risers, but those who are not complain bitterly that life is difficult enough first thing in the morning without the imposition of breakfast. If you cannot face breakfast or haven't got time, do you find yourself nibbling a chocolate bar halfway through the morning or feeling very weak before lunch? Make it a rule for pregnancy that, even if you do not eat breakfast, you will have a nutritious mid-morning snack, for example an orange, some wholemeal bread and an egg (hardboiled if taken to work) or perhaps some muesli and fruit.

If you have to attend the ante-natal clinic 'fasting', try to get an early appointment. Have a bedtime snack the night before and make sure you take something with you to eat as soon as the test has been done (crispbread and cheese or a sandwich).

What you can do about meals which are made for you but not by you
If your weekday lunch meals are provided and there is a choice, opt for plain foods so you can see what you are getting – roast and stewed meats, poultry and fish, simply cooked eggs. Ask for wholemeal bread if it is not on offer – canteen staff can be helpful if they know what you want. Salads may be more nutritious than hot vegetables if these have been finely cut up, soaked in water and then cooked for too long, drained and kept warm. If 'dessert' is not to your fancy, you may be able to get an extra helping of first course, or salad and bread or biscuits and cheese.

If you live in a hostel or for some reason have all your meals prepared for you and they are not to your liking, try lobbying for at least some of the foods you would prefer some of the time. If you buy snacks, choose nuts, wholegrain biscuits, milk, celery, tomatoes, cress, fresh fruit and pure juices. Wheatgerm and bran sprinkled over processed breakfast cereals will boost the vitamin, mineral and fibre content. It may be worth considering a vitamin/mineral supplement or brewer's yeast tablets if the food is poor. Discuss this with your doctor or on your next visit to the ante-natal clinic.

In the case of occasional dining out, what you choose will not matter from a nutritional point of view since you can compensate if necessary by what you eat for the rest of the week. It will matter, however, if you go for a one-time favourite hot spicy dish or rich creamy casserole and then realize to your dismay that it no longer agrees with you in pregnancy. In company, if a choice is available stick to something simple and safe. It can also be difficult if you have to wait ages before eating and everyone else is sipping drinks. Not only do you want to limit or avoid alcohol (see next chapter) but you begin to feel unwell if you don't eat. What about the baby – how does he or she feel? If you choose a fruit or tomato juice, you can make it long-lasting and thirst-quenching by asking for added soda and ice. Do not starve yourself half the day in anticipation of the meal, as you probably did before a special meal when you were

Putting Theory Into Practice

not pregnant. You will feel ill. Plan ahead; have a glass of milk before you leave home and put a small bread roll or a couple of biscuits or a few nuts in clingfilm in your bag or coat pocket. Sneak off to the Ladies Cloakroom for a nibble if you are beginning to wilt and it looks as if a long wait is likely.

In late pregnancy, it may be impossible to manage a several-course meal unless it is very leisurely and lasts for hours. If there is a choice, select 'light' dishes like consommé, fish, and mousse or fruit salad so you will not get over-full. When no choice is available, have a quiet word with the waiter beforehand and ask for smaller portions, or surreptitiously pass on surplus to a hungry neighbour or obliging partner.

FIVE

Nourishing Yourself and Your Baby

It would be wrong to emphasize the value of good food without also recognizing the important influence that other factors can have on the health and well-being of your baby. To nourish means not only to feed but also to cherish and to protect. Cherish yourself by respecting your body's physical and psychological needs for exercise and enjoyment, rest and relaxation. Protect yourself from potential hazards, both environmental and social with the best means at your disposal. Many of these influences which affect your health can interact with nutrition. Some of the factors to be considered here can themselves affect your nutritional status and the effect of others may be modified by the type of food you eat.

Stress

More and more people admit to suffering from stress-related disorders, and stress is part of day-to-day existence for all living things. The human body has sophisticated mechanisms for responding to and dealing with various types of stress – social, psychological or physical. A stress which damages the health of one person may have no effect on another. It is not stress *per se* which causes disease, rather it may be the way the individual responds or the length of time the person is under stress which are the deciding factors.

Why is this relevant to nutrition and to pregnancy? Because body functions interact with each other. A part of the brain called the hypothalamus and the autonomic or involuntary nervous system are involved in responding to stress and they also control such processes as digestion, circulation and reproduction. This is why stress can make you have 'butterflies' in your stomach, goose-pimples, clammy hands or a racing pulse. The body's reactions to the stress of going abroad or leaving home as an adolescent, for example, can be sufficient to cause a disturbance in the normal pattern of menstruation. For men and women, stress can result in an inhibition of sexual arousal or even lead to impotence.

There is some biological foundation for the ideas that prospective parents should be relaxed and not under stress in order to conceive, and that the mother's attitude during pregnancy may be able to be perceived by the baby. Excessive stress can also make you unable to eat or sleep properly, or increase your dependency on coffee, cigarettes or alcohol, and these may undermine your health still further.

So what can you do if you are under excessive stress? Ideally, avoid it, but if you cannot, the only healthful alternative is to increase your capacity to cope. Ways of doing this include taking up hobbies, exercise, relaxation exercises, yoga, meditation and autogenic training. Counselling or group therapy can be helpful to some. If the first thing you try doesn't seem to help much at the beginning, persist for a bit longer and then try something else. Individual problems need individual solutions.

Exercise

Exercise can help with stress, but is also beneficial to health in its own right. Moderate exercise every day is preferable to squash once a week with relative inactivity for the rest of the week.

Before pregnancy, if you have a sedentary job, ways to incorporate more exercise into your daily programme include an early morning exercise programme, a brisk walk in the lunch hour or part of the way to or from work, using stairs instead of lifts; and into your weekly programme, sessions of swimming, tennis, badminton, cycling, hiking, etc. Build up any form of exercise slowly initially or you may do more harm than good.

Those who exercise a great deal, besides needing to eat more, may require extra of certain nutrients, such as vitamin B_2, in their diet. Excessive exercise can produce some unwanted effects – female athletes are more likely to

Eating Well for a Healthy Pregnancy

suffer from amenorrhoea (lack of periods), than less physically active women. Although low body weight can cause the periods to cease for a while, this effect can also occur in women of normal weight who exercise vigorously.

During pregnancy there is no reason why you should not continue to do any exercise to which your body is already accustomed but this is not the time suddenly to start to learn to ride, play squash or do gymnastics. If you normally exercise a lot or have a physically strenuous job and/or a young family, your nutritional requirements may be above average. Avoid over-extending yourself. Trying to cope with a full-time job, jogging, an evening exercise class, cooking and housework could put your developing baby in competition with quite a lot of other demands on your body, and leave little time for essential relaxation.

Rest and relaxation

Pregnancy is not an illness, but nor is it a condition to ignore. Many women are amazed at their need for extra sleep and rest, even during early pregnancy. If you feel very lethargic and want to sleep more than usual, take notice of what your body is signalling to you. Get as much rest as you can, especially if you are sick as well as tired.

The awful tiredness of early pregnancy does not usually last much beyond twelve to fourteen weeks, but even after that, try to have an afternoon rest with your feet up. If you are working, at lunchtime decide what suits you best – a walk or a lie down. An afternoon rest is easier to arrange for those at home on their own, but you have to admit to yourself that it is important. If you already have a toddler who still has a daytime nap, turn a blind eye to any chaos and have a rest yourself at the same time. Unfortunately, lively toddlers can suddenly go off having a nap just when you could really use it. Here are some tactics that may help – lie down on the bed together with a book, settle down in front of a pre-school TV programme or entrust him to an obliging friend if you are lucky enough to have one.

Relaxation classes in preparation for childbirth may be offered at the clinic and/or be available through the National Childbirth Trust (see address list on page 149).

Contraception

The Pill The levels of vitamins and minerals in the blood of women who take oral contraceptives can differ from those of non-users. To give a few examples, vitamin A and copper levels can rise, and vitamin C and zinc levels can go down. However, to assume that the Pill causes deficiencies or excesses of vitamins and minerals is too simplistic a view. Advocates of the Pill proffer an alternative explanation; that the hormones in the Pill cause slight ups and downs in blood levels of nutrients but do not affect body stores, in the same way that the hormones of pregnancy cause blood copper levels to go up during pregnancy without putting the pregnant woman in danger of excess copper.

It is not entirely clear whether Pill users need different amounts of vitamins and minerals from non-users. In one research study of women who took the Pill for more than two-and-a-half years before conception the levels of vitamin B_6 in the umbilical cord at delivery were found to be lower than those of women who did not take the Pill. However, in another investigation the decrease in vitamin B_2 levels usually found in Pill users could be prevented if women ate a diet containing adequate amounts of this vitamin. In still another study, eating plenty of fresh fruit and vegetables obliterated the Pill-associated drop in blood vitamin C. If you have been taking the Pill, a good diet will help to eliminate any adverse effects that the Pill may possibly have had on your nutritional status.

Other concerns about the Pill and pregnancy have centred around the possibility that the Pill might affect fertility or adversely affect the outcome of pregnancy. Some women who have been taking the Pill may take slightly longer to conceive than non-users, but this effect does not appear to be permanent although it could take several months to wear off. The majority of those women who experience a lack of periods after coming off the Pill (post-Pill amenorrhoea) have a good chance of a normal healthy pregnancy eventually, but a few may need to consult a gynaecologist. If you are taking the Pill, it is a good idea to stop for at least three to six months before you try for a baby. Use another form of contraception such as the cap or sheath. This allows time for hormone, vitamin and mineral levels to normalize again, and gives you an opportunity to record the dates of your periods so that when you do become pregnant, the date of birth can be estimated more accurately.

The IUD There appears to be no reason why you should not plan to conceive soon after the removal of an IUD unless you have had special problems such as pelvic inflammatory disease or an ectopic pregnancy associated with IUD use. Heavy periods are sometimes associated with IUD use, and some doctors suggest that it is a good idea to have your iron status checked if you have an IUD and lose a lot of blood. You should also concentrate on eating foods rich in iron and folate, such as liver (see also Chapter 9 for other food sources).

Diseases and disorders

Viruses, bacteria and man have co-existed for thousands of years and the human body has developed a sophisticated defence force, the immune system, which constantly undertakes surveillance, detection and destruction of foreign invaders. Like other body mechanisms, the immune system does not work in isolation. If your nutritional status is good, you are better able to resist or throw off infection. During an infection your body's reserves of nutrients will be depleted, yet your appetite may be poor, so a downward spiral in health can be set in motion. During or after an infection, and as soon as you can eat, concentrate on taking small meals at frequent intervals.

The role of vitamin C in fighting infection is now widely acknowledged, so refortify yourself with vitamin C-rich fruits and vegetables. A vitamin C supplement can ease the symptoms of a heavy cold but it may not be wise to take large doses (of 1 g or 1000 mg or over, sometimes called 'mega'-doses) during pregnancy (see page 129). Codliver oil,

Nourishing Yourself and Your Baby

brewer's yeast and wheatgerm, daily, and some liver and oily fish weekly may aid the process of recovery from an infection. You may feel more hungry for a while until your body is back to normal.

Diseases that might infect an unborn baby
There are some diseases which can infect the baby in the womb and can sometimes cause miscarriage or handicap in the baby. These include rubella (German measles), cytomegalovirus (CMV), toxoplasmosis (an infection which is usually contracted from cats and cat litter), genital herpes and syphilis.

If the mother-to-be catches German measles during the first three months of pregnancy, a termination of the pregnancy may be suggested because there is a twenty to thirty per cent risk that the virus may damage the baby's eyes, ears, heart or brain. After the first three months, the risk of damage is very much less. Before pregnancy you can make sure these risks are avoided by asking your doctor to check your immunity to German measles. If you need to be vaccinated because you are not immune you will be told not to conceive for three months, because a live vaccine is used and there is a small risk that it might harm a baby conceived during that time. Even if you were vaccinated at school ask your doctor to check that you are still immune.

Consult your doctor if you are concerned about any other diseases which might affect an unborn baby. If you or your partner have, or have had, genital herpes or any other genito-urinary disease, and want to remain anonymous, you can make an appointment, be seen and be treated without having to give your name. To do this, phone the nearest General Hospital and ask for the genito-urinary (G.U.) department.

Besides infectious diseases, there are some non-infectious medical disorders (and the drugs used to treat these) which could be potentially harmful to a developing baby. If you have a long-term medical disorder, special care may be necessary to check current health and review treatment, and before pregnancy is the best time to see your doctor about this.

Drugs

The tragically obvious damage caused by thalidomide sharpened our awareness of the possible teratogenic (handicapping) effects of drugs taken during pregnancy. Since that time, the tide of anti-drug feeling has swelled, and fear about drugs during pregnancy has become widespread. This increased awareness of the potential dangers of certain drugs is no bad thing, but it can have undesirable consequences. For some disorders, the illness may be more of a risk to the pregnancy than the drug used to treat it. Also, someone who relies on drug treatment for a longterm medical condition may suddenly stop taking it and rapid withdrawal of that drug may be harmful. If you are on long-term drug therapy for any reason whatsoever, do see your doctor about the best medication for pregnancy, and whether the dose might need to be changed. You will then be able to plan without undue worry.

Whilst there is no doubt that some drugs can be extremely dangerous during pregnancy, the number which have actually been proved to be teratogenic, such as thalidomide, is very small. (There are, however, now some treatments being used in specialist skin clinics which should not be used during pregnancy as they can cause malformations but the drugs used are clearly marked with information.) The use of drugs has increased in the past twenty years but there has been no great increase in the incidence of malformations, although the incidence of lesser degrees of drug-induced damage is not known. Many drugs are not recommended during pregnancy, especially during the early months, not because they are teratogenic or even harmful; rather because they have not been proved with absolute certainty to be safe.

Susceptibility to the harmful effects of a drug may vary enormously between individuals, depending on such factors as genetic make-up or inheritance, and environment (diet, smoking, drinking, pollution). Research with rats indicated that the babies of well-fed rats were little affected by the mother being given thalidomide, but those born to rats given thalidomide *and* on a diet deficient in one of a number of vitamins were much more likely to be damaged. It is the total burden on the mother which counts rather than the individual hazard. In a woman already at risk because she is underweight, eats a very poor diet, and smokes heavily, taking a drug may be the last straw and damage could be done, whereas a well-fed, normal-weight non-smoker may not necessarily be affected.

Nevertheless, the best attitude to adopt in relation to drugs and pregnancy is caution, right from the time you stop using contraceptives, until you have finished breast-feeding. This means caution with all prescribed drugs – whether pills, medicines, lotions, creams or sprays. Before you know you are pregnant the tiny embryo may already be implanted in the womb and vulnerable. In the first three months the baby is particularly sensitive because organs and limbs are forming (see Chapter 1). Even after this some drugs can damage developing tissues. Towards the end of pregnancy certain drugs may make the baby drowsy or unwell for some time after the birth. During breast-feeding drugs may pass into the milk, some may have no effect on the baby but others may be harmful.

Do not accept a prescription from your doctor, and then spend the next few days wondering whether to take it or flush it down the toilet. Mention any fears you have to the doctor before he writes a prescription, and he may either change the medication, or simply reassure you. Consult him too, if you are worried because you have read somewhere or been told that the drug you are taking is harmful in pregnancy. Make an appointment or telephone as soon as you can. Discuss with him both the risks and the benefits. He has at hand, for reference, copious literature on drugs and could also refer to local or national drug information services for the most up to-date information about drugs and pregnancy.

Certain drugs which are not on prescription can be harmful if taken in excessive amounts during pregnancy and/or for prolonged periods. One pill taken occasionally may be all right but avoid taking regularly such drugs as aspirin and other analgesics like codeine, also antacids, laxatives, cough mixtures and similar products which you can buy over the counter at the chemist or in the supermarket. If in doubt, ask the doctor or pharmacist to check up for you.

Coffee and tea (and some soft drinks such as colas) contain the drug caffeine and although it is still controversial whether excessive amounts could be harmful in pregnancy, it is known that caffeine can affect certain nutrients. If you take tea or coffee with a meal, it can inhibit the absorption of iron and may interfere with the way the protein in some foods is used. It would be reasonable to limit coffee and tea consumption to around five mugs a day or less in total and, when feasible, to let an hour elapse between having a meal and drinking either of these.

'Social' drugs such as cannabis are not advisable before or during pregnancy. Specialist advice and treatment is necessary and available for those women who are dependent on narcotic drugs and who are pregnant or contemplating pregnancy.

Smoking

Heavy smoking by the mother can increase the chance that she might have a miscarriage, a smaller baby than average or a baby which dies at the time of birth. Babies born to mothers who smoke heavily are more likely to suffer from chest and ear infections than babies of non-smokers. Effects on the physical and mental development of the baby may persist into later childhood.

How is smoking harmful? Before pregnancy, smoking can damage the blood vessels in the womb, which could later affect placental development. During pregnancy, the carbon monoxide, nicotine and cyanide from cigarettes put the baby at risk. Carbon monoxide combines with the haemoglobin in blood and limits its ability to carry oxygen, so the supply of this important fuel to the baby is reduced. Nicotine decreases the breathing movements the baby makes during its development. It can also decrease the flow of blood in the uterus and placenta and limit the supply of certain nutrients to the baby. Nicotine can also get into the breast milk which could be harmful to the baby after the birth; and it might diminish milk secretion. Cyanide is toxic and in addition can combine with other important nutrients.

As the body tries to get rid of cyanide, vitamin B_{12} is used up.

If you smoke, the battery of facts summarized above may be sufficient incentive to help you to stop. Only you can make the decision. Suppose you accept that smoking is harmful but feel it is better to smoke than batter the toddler, walk out on the family or crumble into depression. Then it may help to get support from a self-help group or ask for help or information at the clinic or surgery, the local Health Education office or write to the Health Education Council. In the meantime try to work out for yourself situations in which you always smoke (after a meal, with a coffee etc) and see if you can substitute completely different activities not normally associated with smoking. Try to find other ways to cope with stress, mentioned on page 71.

When should you stop smoking? The best time of all is from well before you conceive until after you have finished breast-feeding or even for good. Yet it is wrong to think it is too late to do any good if you are already pregnant. Even if some damage has been done, it is never too late for your baby to get some benefit from you stopping smoking. Stop now, completely if you can, but even stopping for a few days at a time will be of some benefit. Your baby will get the equivalent of a breathing space because the haemoglobin in the blood is free to carry its full quota of oxygen again. Stop in the days before the baby is due to be born and you will at least be doing a little bit of good at the time of birth. Smoking is a dangerous hazard for an unborn baby but if you really cannot stop, try in every other respect to swing the balance in your favour. Try *not* to be underweight at the time of conception, gain well during pregnancy, do *not* drink alcohol, and eat the best diet you can with plenty of vitamin C-rich foods, since smoking increases your need for this vitamin.

Alcohol

Whether it be a wedding, christening, dinner party, just an evening out or the smallest of celebrations, it would be unusual and for many a gloomy occasion without alcohol.

Eating Well for a Healthy Pregnancy

For centuries alcohol has been an integral part of the social framework of most cultures. So too have been the warnings about the dangers of alcohol in pregnancy. These span from biblical times when the mother of Samson was counselled to give up wine in pregnancy, right up to the present day. The term fetal alcohol syndrome (FAS) was coined to describe the children born to some alcoholic mothers – children whose growth is retarded, who have abnormalities of the face, limbs and heart, who fail to thrive, are mentally deficient and have poor muscle co-ordination.

There is no doubt that alcoholism can seriously damage the unborn child but there is still doubt over exactly how much alcohol is dangerous and how much, if any, is safe. It is now evident that even moderate amounts of alcohol may be harmful to some pregnant women. Studies in America found that women who drank daily had an increased incidence of miscarriage; in France, women drinking more than 400 ml (40 cl or 0.4 l) of wine daily, increased the risk of a low birthweight baby or a stillbirth; and in London studies showed that drinking more than ten drinks weekly before as well as during pregnancy doubled the risk of a low birthweight baby, when compared to having less than five drinks weekly. (One drink equals ½ pint of beer, or one 4 oz glass of wine, or one measure of spirits). The type of drink makes no difference – it is the total amount of alcohol consumed which matters. One woman may be able to drink every day throughout pregnancy with no apparent ill effect, another may be putting her baby at risk of alcohol-related damage, even though she drinks less. The effect of alcohol is unpredictable. Other risk factors such as smoking, poor diet and being underweight may increase susceptibility to alcohol damage. Smoking certainly makes things worse so that women who smoke *and* drink are increasing the risks much more.

When is the baby most vulnerable? At almost every stage of pregnancy and even before conception. During the period after ovulation the egg or ovum may be at risk. Heavy drinking around the time of conception may be especially damaging; the tiny embryo can easily be killed or the baby miscarried a few weeks later. Excess alcohol in early pregnancy could cause malformations. These can vary from the whole range of fetal alcohol problems to a single developmental weakness, such as a heart defect. This could be caused by just one really heavy bout of drinking at a critical stage of heart development. From twelve to eighteen weeks and in the last three months of pregnancy, alcohol may affect brain cell development and subsequent behaviour after birth.

What you can do to protect your baby
1. The safest policy of all is no alcohol before and during pregnancy. (If you are embarrassed about not drinking at a social gathering, have a mixer – tonic or ginger etc. and no one will know there is no spirit in it.) However, one glass of wine, sherry, spirits or beer taken occasionally during pregnancy is not known to cause damage. If you must drink, preferably limit it to one drink a day (or at the most 2 drinks on any one day), and restrict your weekly intake to five drinks or less.

2. At all costs, avoid any situation where you may get drunk or have a binge. One single heavy session could be just as dangerous as heavy drinking regularly.

3. If you do drink regularly and have previously had a miscarriage, complication of pregnancy or a low birth-weight baby, it is worth giving serious thought to abstaining completely from alcohol for the months before and during pregnancy.

4. If you are on any medication, check with your doctor beforehand whether it is safe to take any alcohol at all.

5. Alcohol can pass into breast milk and make the baby drowsy. The occasional glass of beer, stout or wine for a harassed nursing mother may save the day and settle both her and the baby but it is probably best not to exceed one drink daily.

Pollution

Excessive machinery noise, chemical hazards, anaesthetic gases or radiation can pollute you at work; lead in your water or additives in your food can pollute you at home; oil

Eating Well for a Healthy Pregnancy

on the beach or industrial discharges in the sea can pollute you on holiday. Pollution is all around us. Yet you need to keep a sense of proportion by seeing such hazards not in isolation but in relation to everything else you do. Balance today's hazards with benefits. Two hundred years ago environmental hazards to health were no less; they were just different.

We are very much at the mercy of national and commercial bodies for the surveillance of hazards at work and pollutants in water and food. At present each individual also has to take some responsibility for limiting his or her exposure to such hazards and for minimizing personal susceptibility by maintaining good health and eating good food.

If you are not using contraceptives and there is even a remote possibility that you could be pregnant, avoid any x-ray of hips, abdomen or lower back. Check your exposure if you work with radiation. Modern scavenging equipment in operating theatres reduces the risk of damage to the embryo caused by lengthy exposure to anaesthetic gases. It has been suggested, but in many cases not proved, that certain industrial chemicals might increase the risk of menstrual problems and infertility, miscarriage, and growth-retarded or malformed babies. There is also some concern that working in laboratories or in industries involved with rubber, plastics, viscose rayon, smelting, printing, soldering, painting, electronics and motor vehicle repair could constitute a reproductive hazard but a great deal more research is still needed to find out if the few early reports can be substantiated.

You may not feel that you are in a position to do very much about it, short of giving up your job, but you can. Start, if possible, before you become pregnant. Ask your employer and safety representative if there are any substances which may be a reproductive hazard. Consult reference books (see reading list on page 144), or the local Health and Safety Executive (in the phone book). Your doctor may be able to obtain up-to-date reports from a local or national poisons information service. Where there are established safety procedures at work, take special care to observe them.

Reduce the risk from other factors which could make you

more vulnerable, such as smoking or drinking. Protect yourself with a good diet – as an example of just how important diet is, it has been found that individuals who were exposed to the same amount of lead, absorbed quite different amounts from the digestive system into their body, depending on the food they ate. Those with a low dietary intake of 'friendly' minerals such as iron, copper and zinc absorbed a greater amount of lead than did those eating a diet containing adequate amounts of the protective minerals. In Chapter 9, there is a table listing food sources of these minerals.

Besides lead, pollutants in and on the food you eat can come to you as a result of current agricultural and food manufacturing processes and practices. Cereals and vegetables, unless organically grown, may contain traces of insecticides, pesticides or other chemicals and may be passed on to humans either directly or indirectly after passage through cows, pigs, sheep or poultry. In desperation, and with little justification, some people become vegetarian, believing plant food may be less polluted; others peel all fruits and vegetables in the hope of removing pollutants; others do not eat liver for fear that it may have accumulated toxins. The list could go on. The choice is yours. Weigh up both the pros and cons. Limiting your diet could have the opposite effect to that intended – vegetables can be polluted too, and as the skins of vegetables and fruit are removed some of the vitamins and minerals may be peeled away. An increasing number of scientists believe that the best action is positive – to concentrate on eating plenty of the protective substances, whether of plant or animal origin, such as those in wholegrains, vegetables, fruits and liver and let these take care of any 'anti' nutrients; and to wash all fruit and vegetables thoroughly.

While it has not been conclusively proved that food colourings, anti-oxidants, preservatives etc. added during food processing, can damage a fetus, it makes sense not to overload your system with such substances, especially since many foods containing a lot of additives are also highly refined and processed and may have been depleted of vitamins and minerals. Read the food labels if you are interested in avoiding additives.

SIX

When It's Not So Easy

It is often assumed that women 'bloom' during pregnancy so it can come as rather a let-down if you feel other than radiant. Yet large numbers of pregnant women are affected by the so-called 'minor' disorders of pregnancy. Although not usually harmful to the pregnancy, such problems can make life a misery for some women for weeks or possibly even for months on end. This chapter deals with some of the problems which can be alleviated by nutritional means.

Pregnancy sickness

Even the most determined resolution to nourish yourself well can be broken in the first few weeks of pregnancy, all because of something usually labelled a 'minor complaint' – namely, nausea and vomiting. If you are pregnant and sick, you may feel you are the only pregnant woman who could possibly be feeling so miserable. Yet what you are experiencing is almost as common as pregnancy itself: approximately three-quarters of all pregnant women have some form of sickness. Knowing that someone somewhere will be feeling just as bad as you, and that sickness is part of normal pregnancy for many women, will not make the sickness go away but it may help you to tolerate it a bit more easily.

Pregnancy sickness may cause other temporary problems. If you have other young children they may not be able to understand your sudden apparent decline in health and temperament. Your partner may feel powerless to help, and worry also that he will suffer setbacks at work if he has to take time off to look after you or the family. Unless he knows someone else whose wife has suffered similarly he may even begin to wonder if you are exaggerating your symptoms. If you are single, you may be without emotional and practical support and under pressure to conceal your pregnancy from others.

All too often, whether it comes from a book or magazine,

When It's Not So Easy

a doctor or a friend, advice about pregnancy pays scant attention to the problem of pregnancy sickness. So this chapter is mainly about coping with sickness, what symptoms you may have, and why it is that you feel so awful. Hopefully, it will reassure you to see the symptoms written down and, if need be, may help you to convince others that your suffering is real. The sympathy, understanding and practical support of relatives and friends can be a great help to you. If you are not seriously troubled by sickness you may prefer to skip the next section.

Symptoms

'Morning' sickness is not an appropriate description, since less than one tenth of women are sick in the early morning only. The sickness can range from occasional mild nausea to severe nausea and vomiting which goes on all day, every day and even during the night, or even to a condition known as hyperemesis gravidarum (very severe sickness), when hospital treatment is needed.

Nausea can be the worst symptom, especially if it persists throughout your waking hours. It becomes more extreme on an empty stomach and can make you retch. The dreadful thing about retching is that you feel that you want to be very, very sick but your violent efforts to be so may bring little or no relief.

The urge to vomit can occur in the middle of a meal or immediately after eating, and the onset can be so sudden that you may have no warning. Quite unlike other forms of sickness when you do not feel like food for some time afterwards, you may find that you feel much better straight away and want to eat. While actually eating, you may feel blissfully free from sickness only to find the symptoms return shortly afterwards. This can lead to endless nibbling in order to keep the nausea at bay.

Unexpected changes in weight can occur in the early months. If your appetite is insatiable, or you have mild nausea and find food the best form of relief, you may find your clothes begin to get tight very soon. However, when these symptoms subside, your pattern of weight gain should balance out. On the other hand, if you have severe sickness and are losing weight, you may worry that your baby might suffer. There is no evidence that this would happen, and providing you were in good health and eating well before you became pregnant, your body reserves will be able to cope with this period (see page 4). However, if you lose more than a half a stone, consult your doctor and mention it at the clinic when you go for an appointment.

Pregnancy sickness can be exhausting and you may also have to cope with the physical tiredness which affects so many pregnant women, whether they are sick or not. This is not something you can shrug off and snap out of, but try to rest whenever you can so that you do not get too overtired as this can aggravate the sickness.

Causes of sickness

Little is known about exactly what causes sickness in pregnancy. One reason the subject has received low priority for research may be because it appears to have no harmful longterm effects, on either you or the baby. Indeed, traditionally, pregnancy sickness is seen as a good sign. On the other hand, if you are not sick, this does not mean that something is wrong; it may be that you are one of the lucky women whose body adapts more readily to the pregnant condition.

There have been several theories about what causes pregnancy sickness. One of these relates to the hormone hCG (human chorionic gonadotrophin). This special pregnancy hormone begins to circulate in your blood a few days after you conceive. More and more is produced until a peak is reached around nine to ten weeks after your last menstrual period. Quite a lot of this hormone passes out into your urine; and it is the presence of this hormone which makes your pregnancy test positive. The quantity of hCG circulating round your body usually drops dramatically some time after twelve weeks. The high levels of hCG usually coincide with the time when pregnancy sickness is at its worst, and consequently this hormone has been linked with pregnancy sickness. This seems a reasonable explanation but it has not yet been proved and other hormones have at one time or another been thought to be involved.

A nutritionally related reason for pregnancy sickness is another possibility. As early as the 1920s it was suggested that women with more severe forms of sickness were likely to report that they were accustomed to a high protein, low carbohydrate diet. A high carbohydrate diet was found to be very helpful and even today carbohydrate-rich foods such as bread, cereals and potatoes are recommended to relieve the sickness. Preliminary findings in more recent research showing that some women suffering from severe sickness may have taken slightly more protein in their usual diet before pregnancy than do women with little or no sickness, are now being followed up.

In the 1940s, vitamin B_6 was tried and found to be helpful for treating pregnancy sickness. The body's need for this vitamin does seem to increase during pregnancy and it could be that women with severe pregnancy sickness either cannot obtain sufficient vitamin B_6 from their food or have an unusually high requirement for this vitamin in pregnancy. So far, however, it would seem that although dietary habits may contribute to the nausea and vomiting, they probably play only a small part and many other factors must be involved.

'If you're very sick, there's more chance that your baby will be a girl', – like many other old wives' tales, this may have a grain of truth in it. Women taken into hospital with very severe sickness seem to have a *slightly* greater than usual chance of having a girl. For example, records have shown that, of 659 women admitted to hospital with hyperemesis, 307 gave birth to boys and 352 to girls.

Pregnancy sickness was at one time considered to be a psychological disturbance. Research did not confirm this and this view is no longer widely held but some sick women still find themselves regarded as emotionally unable to cope with such a minor 'feminine' complaint. This attitude is completely unjustified. However, when sickness is extremely severe, some doctors consider that psychological problems may be adding to the distress. As can happen with so many other illnesses, any extra stress such as moving house, bereavement, a change of shift work, unhappiness or lack of sleep can aggravate the symptoms.

What you can do
Try to accept the sickness and not feel guilty if you don't

Eating Well for a Healthy Pregnancy

want to do anything, see anyone or cook proper meals. These feelings will pass. If you can talk to someone who has suffered similarly, she may have some useful tips and you can be sure of having a sympathetic ear. Some find companionship can be very therapeutic – you may find you don't vomit so much in your neighbour's house or when you are with visitors.

Fresh air can help, even if it is only for a short time during a lunch hour or when taking a child out for a walk. Bending and stretching may make matters worse, so do not worry if jobs around the house do not get done. It does help to rest as much as possible. Whether you are at work or caring for a toddler, try to take frequent rests with your feet up during the day. You may feel the need to go to bed very early – 6 or 8 o'clock. Wear loose clothing around your middle and try a hot-water bottle for relief.

Mild to moderate sickness For those with mild to moderate sickness, the nausea usually gets worse on an empty stomach so eating little and often may work better than trying to tackle large regular meals. If a main meal can be managed, it is usually better to take this in the middle of the day rather than in the evening. Keep to a balanced diet if possible or try to eat nutritious foods like wholemeal bread or wholegrain cereals, potatoes and fruit rather than biscuits and cakes.

This may be easier said than done and you may not be able to face the more wholesome foods. A lot of women can only manage white bread, perhaps because their digestive system is more sluggish than usual. Any food is better than no food – it is better to take something less nutritious which will stay down rather than to take nothing at all and find the sickness getting progressively worse. So during this time eat what you can face – odd food fads will not matter for a few weeks as long as you eat a balanced diet over the rest of your pregnancy.

There are no hard and fast rules about what foods are most helpful as each woman differs and has to try and find what suits her best. The following is just a guide to the type of eating pattern which may be helpful.

When It's Not So Easy

- ☐ *On awakening*
  Dry toast, crackers or biscuits (eat these slowly before you even sit up in bed and wait a few minutes before getting up).
- ☐ *Breakfast*
  Porridge or other cereal.
  Stewed apples, prunes or other fruit.
  Toast with honey, marmalade, jam or yeast extract.
- ☐ *Mid-morning*
  Toast or sandwich, crackers or biscuit, or a few nuts.
- ☐ *Lunchtime*
  Soup.
  An egg, meat or fish as sandwiches or with bread, crackers or pasta (plain spaghetti or macaroni).
  Fruit, custard or ice cream.
- ☐ *Mid-afternoon*
  Toast, cracker or biscuit.
  Fruit or nuts.
- ☐ *Late-afternoon*
  Bread or toast with yeast extract, jam or honey.
  Biscuit or cake.
- ☐ *Dinner*
  Small portion of main meal if wanted, for example: mashed potato and vegetable, small portion of fish or chicken or meat.
  Dessert of rice, sago, semolina pudding, fruit or raisins.
- ☐ *Mid-evening*
  Dry toast, cracker, biscuit or nuts.
- ☐ *Bedtime*
  Cereal and milk, toast or banana sandwich.
  (You may not feel like a snack at this time but it will help to lessen the nausea first thing in the morning.)
- ☐ *During the night*
  Keep dry biscuits, a bun or fruit and a drink by your bed in case you wake up feeling sick.

Fit in your drinks either with or between meals, whichever you prefer. Although many people frown on the use of sugar, honey, etc., sweetened drinks can prove helpful during the period when you are sick. Try adding glucose instead of sugar if you do not like the sweet taste.

When travelling or shopping, have something handy to suck or chew to help avoid vomiting, e.g. glucose sweets, barley sugars, mints, fruit gums or caramels. Although these are not nutritious they can be very useful in emergencies. A tried and tested remedy for travel sickness is ginger, so try sucking tiny pieces of crystallized ginger (from health food shop or specialist grocer).

Women taking part in surveys on pregnancy sickness have contributed suggestions about which foods they found helpful. Some of these are given below as ideas to try:

☐ *Drinks*
   Yeast extract in hot water.
   Fizzy drinks, e.g. lemonade, ginger ale, soda water.
   Plain water. Mineral water.
   Ginger 'tea' (pour boiling water on to crushed root ginger and leave to brew. Sweeten to taste).
   Ice-cold milk or hot milky drinks.
   Pure fruit juices: orange, grapefruit, apple, lemon, pineapple. Alone or diluted with water or soda water.
   Weak tea (with or without milk, sugar or lemon).
   Dilutable drinks: lemon and lime, lemon barley water etc.

☐ *Meat and alternatives*
   Plainly cooked meat and poultry. Eggs lightly boiled, poached, scrambled or as egg custard. Fish poached or steamed in milk. Hazelnuts, almonds. Pulses simply cooked.

☐ *Bread and cereals*
   Bread plain, toasted or as sandwiches. If fats upset you, try other spreads such as jam, marmalade, honey or yeast extract. There is no need to eat hot meals if you do not want them, and sandwiches can form a simply prepared meal: try egg, tomato, salad, banana, cold chicken, tongue or other cold meat.
   Breakfast cereals e.g. porridge, muesli, gruel (add 2 tablespoons of medium oatmeal to 1 pint cold water. Stir occasionally and leave overnight. Stir again, sieve off oatmeal and discard these. Boil up remaining liquid

until it thickens and reduces in volume by about half. Surplus can be kept in the fridge for a day or two. When ready to drink, heat and add salt, sugar, lemon juice and/or milk to taste.)

Biscuits: wholemeal ones such as crispbread or digestives may be better for you, but others such as cream crackers, rich tea, gingernuts, baby rusks, may also help.

Rice and pasta: rice, sago, semolina, spaghetti or macaroni (avoid having a rich sauce with it).

☐ *Fruit and vegetables*

If you can take fruit, try sucking slices of fresh orange, grapefruit, or tangerine. Crisp apples or stewed apples, grapes, bananas, prunes or dried fruit can help.

Some women find certain vegetables helpful: tomatoes (in sandwiches), raw carrots, celery, mushy peas, mashed carrots. Try potatoes mashed, boiled or baked in jackets.

Smooth mild flavoured soups are best and if you cannot face making your own, try tinned cream soups such as tomato, mushroom.

☐ *Milk and milk products*

If you cannot manage milk by itself, try with cereals or in mashed potatoes, rice pudding or custard.

Cheese: devotees often go right off it, whilst others may find it tolerable.

Severe sickness If the sickness is very severe, go to bed if possible. Lying down and staying still and quiet, even while trying to keep nibbling and drinking, helps reduce vomiting. Keep eating and drinking separate. If at certain times of the day, nothing you try seems to stay down, let your stomach rest during this period. There may be another time when some foods will stay down and small snacks of, for example, poached egg, a few nuts, or some cereal, should be tried then.

It will be a great help if your partner or a neighbour can take over in the kitchen when you are at your worst, and bring you small snacks on a tray into another room. You will probably not feel at all like getting food for yourself

Eating Well for a Healthy Pregnancy

(even the thought of it may start you retching) but if you go without food or drink you will most likely get worse. It is worth at least a try to have a drink of water or milk and be sick, and then try eating a small meal. Having something to be sick on may make your stomach less sore than continual retching on an empty stomach.

If you really cannot eat, try taking small sips of a drink or you may become dehydrated and ill. Add one teaspoon of powdered glucose (from chemists) and a pinch of bicarbonate of soda to a mug of warm water or any other drink you can manage, and keep sipping very slowly.

If the sickness is really bad, do not hesitate to call your doctor. He may not want to recommend anything other than a dry biscuit and a cup of tea in bed but he will be able to reassure you that everything is all right. Alternatively, he may prescribe a tried and tested drug because he feels it is justified in your particular circumstances.

Some people recommend taking a supplement of vitamin B_6 as this has been used for a long time for treating pregnancy sickness. Discuss this possibility with your doctor. The pill sizes are usually 10, 20, 50 or 100 mg. It may be helpful in moderate doses (20–100 mg a day). You can also take foods which are high in vitamin B_6 such as cereals, banana, yeast extract, wheatgerm and brewer's yeast. Do not take *any* drugs or medicines for sickness without asking your doctor if they are safe to take during pregnancy. In fact, you should even tell your doctor if you are thinking of buying your own vitamin B_6 (pyridoxine) from the chemist.

Finally, be assured that it will get better eventually. Even if the sickness lasts longer than you expect, hang on to the fact that, at worst, it cannot last longer than nine months. You will be surprised how soon you forget it once the sickness stops and you have a lovely baby. In the meantime, try to think of yourself as coasting along, slowly getting through one day at a time and diverting yourself as much as possible with TV, magazines, books, knitting, etc.

Cravings and aversions

Whether sick or not, many women have various aversions or odd food cravings during pregnancy (although it is just as

When It's Not So Easy

normal not to have cravings as it is to have them). Examples of foods commonly avoided include meat, fatty and spicy foods, rich sauces and drinks such as tea, coffee and alcohol. There are always exceptions, of course – for example, Deirdre could not manage without her daily plate of chips. Cravings are often for starchy foods such as white bread, cakes and potatoes. Joanna admitted to buying and eating a whole loaf of crusty white bread in one go. She could not even resist starting it as soon as she left the shop.

Many women have commented about this almost irresistible urge in connection with a particular food. Fruit or pickles are a favourite with some. Julie seemed unable to quench her desire for satsumas, yet Lesley could not so much as look at an orange without turning green. The symptom of pica (a craving for a non-food substance such as coal), is fairly unusual nowadays but if you have it try not to worry – it will pass. Imelda confessed to crunching sand from the children's sandpit and was very relieved when this strange craving disappeared after her baby was born.

A nasty metallic taste in the mouth can often occur in the early months and a few women experience the problem of ptyalism (too much saliva). This is thought to occur because the part of the brain involved with nausea and vomiting is very close to that involved with controlling saliva production, and swallowing the saliva you normally produce suddenly becomes more difficult or almost impossible. It is not a serious health problem though it may make you utterly miserable. You can save yourself embarrassment by keeping an ample supply of hankies or paper towels at the ready.

Your sense of smell can often seem more acute during pregnancy. Petrol fumes, perfume, disinfectants and aromas from the kitchen or wafting down the street from a cafe, may become intolerable. Conversely, you may find you have an obsession to sniff repeatedly a particular fragrance or odour. Wendy, for example, would walk all over town to find road-workers laying down new tarmac, so that she could stand and sniff the smell of new tar.

Constipation

Constipation is very common during pregnancy and is thought to occur because the hormones of pregnancy have a relaxing effect on the bowel muscles, so that they work less efficiently than usual. In addition, the enlarging womb is exerting more pressure which can make matters worse. Quite often the iron tablets which you may have been given can aggravate the problem. Some women suffer from haemorrhoids or 'piles' and these can cause discomfort, burning and itching.

Again, there are several dietary measures which can help. These include drinking more, and eating more high-fibre foods such as wholemeal bread, wholegrain cereals, fruits and vegetables (for example, baked potatoes in their jackets, cabbage), dried fruits (especially prunes and figs which have a natural laxative effect). Adding one or two teaspoons of unprocessed bran to your breakfast cereal can help but do not use large amounts of extra bran regularly, especially if you are a vegetarian. Too much bran could interfere with the absorption of minerals from your food.

Laxatives should be avoided unless absolutely necessary, and even then consult your doctor before taking anything. Very strong laxatives may stimulate the uterus to contract. Some doctors recommend that laxatives containing liquid paraffin should not be used regularly because the absorption of vitamins A and D could be adversely affected. Preparations based on natural products or bulking agents are often recommended.

Heartburn

Heartburn has nothing to do with your heart; it is called heartburn simply because it feels as if it is near to your heart. Most women usually think of heartburn as something which can occur later in pregnancy because of the upward pressure of the enlarging baby, so it can come as a surprise to find yourself experiencing this in early pregnancy. The reason is that this problem, like that of constipation, is thought to be caused by the relaxing effect

When It's Not So Easy

of some of the pregnancy hormones on the muscles of the digestive system. It becomes easier for the normal acid contents of the stomach to come back up into your oesophagus (the tube connecting your mouth to your stomach), causing a burning sensation there.

Treatments are usually intended to prevent or counteract the acid coming up into your oesophagus. It is commonly recommended that you sleep propped up on several pillows and that whenever possible you sit with a straight back. Try to avoid bending, straining and constipation, as these may all aggravate the symptoms. It is advisable to avoid large meals – so divide up the day's food into a number of small meals. Have your last meal an hour or two before going to bed. In addition, it is worth trying to relax at mealtimes, eat slowly and chew your food well. If the heartburn is still very severe despite all your efforts to treat it, do see your doctor or mention it at the ante-natal clinic. You may be prescribed an antacid, or an alternative preparation, but medicines like these should only be taken under medical supervision.

Leg cramps

Despite the commonly held opinion that calcium salts will cure nocturnal leg cramps during pregnancy, this has not been proven. If you are advised to take extra calcium and this helps, carry on. If it does not, it may be worth trying a little extra salt in your daily diet, since there is some evidence that this can help. During an attack try stretching the affected muscles and massaging them.

SEVEN

Special Needs

Pregnancy is a special time for all women who have babies, but there are some women whose needs are increased above the average or whose needs are different from those of most pregnant women. Examples include women pregnant in their teens or in their later years, vegans, women having twins, women with a food allergy or a medical condition such as diabetes. Women who have previously experienced anaemia or pre-eclampsia in pregnancy and those for whom an earlier pregnancy failed, perhaps because of a miscarriage or stillbirth, also have special needs. These can be dealt with only briefly here. If you need to know more, refer to the follow-up reading and address lists (pages 145–50) and ask your doctor's advice about any special medical care which may be necessary.

Very young or older mothers-to-be

A girl under sixteen needs special care in pregnancy largely because her own growth and development are not complete and so her own extra nutritional needs are added to those of pregnancy. It has been suggested that teenagers who are still growing may need to gain more weight than older women during pregnancy. The older teenager is, in theory, at an ideal biological age for pregnancy but her potential can be severely undermined by obsessions about body image and weight, irregular eating habits, poor choice of food, living away from home, financial or psychological problems.

The older mother-to-be nowadays has excellent prospects if she has good medical care and personal attention to health. However, there are one or two problems which can be associated with being an older parent. It may take slightly longer for you to conceive. Fecundity may begin to decline slightly after the age of thirty and markedly after the age of

Special Needs

thirty-five. Even if there is nothing wrong in reproductive terms, this delay can cause anxiety, which in itself might inhibit conception. Where there is a real problem of subfertility, either in the man or the woman, if you are older it leaves fewer years for a chance to conceive, should medical help be needed. It is known that the incidence of Down's syndrome (mongolism) increases with age but this can now be detected by the amniocentesis test in which a sample of amniotic fluid is taken from the womb. A termination is offered if necessary. The experiences of many other first-time mothers have been documented in *Birth over Thirty* by Sheila Kitzinger (see reading list on page 145).

Records show that the age range of twenty to thirty is the best in which to have a baby, since it is associated with the greatest likelihood of a healthy outcome. If you can, plan to have your first baby while you are in this age group but if this is not possible and you are a younger or older mother-to-be, focus on those factors which you can do something about. Pay special attention to eating good food and maintaining the right weight for you, as already described (see page 38). Avoid all habits and hazards which may jeopardize your chances of having a healthy baby.

Mothers carrying twins

It makes sense to eat more if you are carrying twins. Double check your diet and add more protein and calories to the basic diet for pregnancy. An easy way to do this is to add an extra pint of milk a day plus a little more from the meat and alternatives group (see page 17). If the thought of two pints of milk daily appals you, instead have an extra meal containing a portion from the meat and alternatives group or increase the serving size of your ordinary meals, for example 6 oz meat instead of 3–4 oz.

Canadian studies have shown that women carrying twins who eat well and gain proportionately more weight have healthy babies and a very low chance of experiencing the medical condition pre-eclampsia (see page 106) in pregnancy – and they do regain their figures afterwards. In fact, one woman even gained 80 lb in pregnancy. She gave birth to babies weighing over 7 lb each, and was back to her normal weight six months after the birth!

As pregnancy progresses, your increased size will make it difficult to eat three main meals – little and often is more attractive and essential. Nuts and raisins, cheese and apple, cereal and milk, banana and wholemeal bread make good between-meal snacks. The nutritional demands on you will increase still further during breast-feeding so don't feel guilty if you have a monumental appetite. Rest is doubly important too, both during pregnancy and whilst breast-feeding. Because you have double the work, you may need help from relations and friends. Also discuss with your doctor the possibility of a home help.

If you are carrying more than twins, then add an extra food allowance for each extra baby!

Vegetarians/vegans

If you are a vegetarian or vegan, your needs are just the same as those of anyone else who becomes pregnant. These can be met by careful choice within the framework of your type of diet. However, being a vegan or vegetarian does not confer on you some magical protection from nutritional inadequacy. Your diet is still only as good as you choose to make it.

The four food group system already described (see page 16) easily fits in with a lacto-vegetarian diet. The vegan mother-to-be, however, may find she is accused of neglecting her own and her baby's needs for various nutrients such as protein, vitamin B_{12} and minerals.

Most well-balanced diets in the West contain more than enough protein but vegans may need to take a little extra care over this during pregnancy. Beans, peas, lentils and soy products are good sources of protein. The proteins in all foods are made up of a mixture of amino acids (sub-units which make proteins) and vegetable protein sources may be deficient in one or other of the so-called essential amino acids. Although it is now recognized that the 'complementary' mixing of different protein sources (to ensure that all the amino acids are present) is not essential at *every* meal for most vegans, it may still be advisable during pregnancy.

Special Needs

Vitamin B_{12} is found only in animal foods and some nutritionists recommend that vegans take a B_{12} supplement – but do check with your doctor first.

It has been argued that vegetarians and vegans are more at risk of low mineral status because minerals are not as readily available from plant foods and substances called oxalates, tannates and phytates, which may inhibit mineral absorption, are present in some vegetables. However, other research has shown that blood mineral levels of healthy vegetarians are within the normal range. So undue concern is not warranted, unless laboratory tests have shown that you have a nutritional deficiency or you do not feel or look very well. This can happen if the choice of vegetarian foods is inadequate but if you are a vegan and you choose carefully what to eat for pregnancy, you can prove the critics wrong.

Check the points given below and, if you can, begin this eating plan several months before pregnancy:

1. If you have become thin on a vegetarian diet, try to increase your weight into the normal range as described in Chapter 3. This may mean eating more, and more often, and increasing your intake of protein and high calorie foods, as described below.

2. Adapt the four food group scheme (see page 26) to suit a vegan diet. Substitute soy milk and soy products for the milk and milk products group (4 cups soy milk daily or equivalent). Take two large or three small servings from the pulses, nuts and seeds group. Many vegan recipes already mix the different complementary protein sources; examples include:

☐ cereals (rice, barley, wheat) + pulses (peas, beans, lentils)
   e.g. baked beans on wholemeal toast.

☐ soy products + seeds + cereals
   e.g. tempeh with tahini sauce and vegetables served with rice; bread made with wheat and soy flour and sesame seeds.

☐ seeds + pulses
   e.g. chick peas and tahini (hummus)
   casseroles and soups with sesame and beans.

Cereal foods are also sources of protein, so vegans should take extra portions (6-7 helpings daily) to make up the protein requirement. In the vegetable and fruit group, add to the recommended amounts, 2 extra portions of vitamin C-rich fruit and vegetables, an extra portion of dark green vegetables and also a carotene-rich food.

3. Some of the ways to make sure you get enough iron (and other minerals) for both you and the baby are:

a) Eat iron-rich foods daily (e.g. figs, prunes and prune juice, apricots and other dried fruit, molasses, brewer's yeast, cocoa). Although wheatgerm, lentils and spinach contain good quantities of iron, its availability is limited by the other substances present. Vegetables such as potatoes, beetroot, broccoli, tomato, cauliflower, and cabbage may be better sources of iron because they contain less of inhibitory substances and more of substances such as vitamin C which aid absorption.

b) Vitamin C enhances the absorption of iron from plant foods. Take advantage of this and eat vitamin C-rich vegetables and fruit with food sources of iron – orange with your breakfast cereal, salads and vegetables with your main pulse/seed meals.

c) Tea and coffee taken with a meal can inhibit iron absorption (and may affect protein availability) so when convenient, try to have any tea or coffee one hour or more after a meal.

d) If you have an iron frying pan, use it often for cooking. This will add extra traces of iron to your food. However, iron from the pan can destroy vitamin C during cooking, so cook vitamin C-rich vegetables in non-iron pans.

e) Check Chapter 9 on vitamins and minerals for good sources of minerals from vegetable foods.

4. Extra calories are needed for pregnancy, and even after you have included the protein foods and the other food groups, it may be difficult to eat enough bulk to supply these calories, so energy-dense foods should be included – foods rich in oils and fats, such as nuts, coconut, peanuts, chocolate, olives, vegetable oils and salad dressings.

Special Needs

If you are in any doubt about your health and diet, ask your doctor if you need blood tests to assess your vitamin and mineral status and if you can see a dietitian to go over the diet you usually eat. Get further information about vegan diets from books in the reading list on page 145 and contact the Vegan and Vegetarian Societies (see page 150).

Food allergy or intolerances and pregnancy

The proliferation of theories to explain food allergy or intolerances – inheritance, bottle feeding, deficient diets, toxins, food additives, to name a few, has been paralleled by the growing list of foods blamed for causing allergy. Yet food allergy is not new – 'One man's meat is another man's poison' is a quotation at least 2000 years old.

Strictly speaking, food *allergy* is an adverse reaction by the body which involves the immune or defence system. Other unpleasant responses to food are often described as food *intolerances*. Common foods to which some susceptible people are allergic include milk, eggs and wheat-based foods. This is not because there is anything inherently wrong with these foods but merely that they are commonly eaten. In different countries with different dietary habits, other foods will be top of the list for causing allergy. The order of foods in the league table can change if dietary habits change. For example, allergy to soy products is on the increase in this country, because more soy-based foods are being eaten.

Food intolerances can range from minor ones which are uncomfortable to those which are potentially dangerous and life-threatening. They can be inborn or develop gradually. For instance, lactose intolerance develops when a person gradually loses the ability to digest the lactose in milk. If milk and dairy products must be avoided, considerable care is needed to ensure that the many prepared and processed foods which can contain milk are avoided too. Further attention is needed to ensure that calcium needs for pregnancy and lactation are adequately met.

If you are pregnant or thinking of becoming pregnant and have a food allergy or intolerance, seek professional advice as early as possible. Do not attempt to diagnose and treat allergy by yourself – you may be needlessly limiting your diet. Detailed tests carried out on people who had been avoiding a particular food or foods thinking they were allergic, showed that quite a proportion were not allergic. Their allergy was imagined.

If, however, you really are allergic, and the guilty food(s) is (are) a common constituent(s) of the average daily diet, it may not be easy to plan a varied and nutritious diet for pregnancy without it (them) but it can be done. Dietitians are quite familiar with devising special menus, recipes and shopping lists. Supplements may be recommended in certain cases under medical supervision. Self-help groups are springing up as, too, is the range of books on the subject.

Diabetes and pregnancy

There is a difference between the diabetic person who becomes pregnant and the pregnant woman who becomes diabetic.

For *the long-term insulin-dependent diabetic*, it is essential that specialist medical care and attention starts well before conception and continues right through pregnancy. Consult your doctor and diabetes specialist about this.

The diabetes which can develop during pregnancy is called gestational diabetes and usually disappears after the birth. You may find that modern treatments for gestational diabetes include a diet rich in fibre from wholesome foods because it seems that this can be beneficial.

If something has gone wrong in the past in relation to pregnancy

Infertility and subfertility
One of the most tragic things of all when a couple desperately want to have children is for there to be no pregnancy at all. Many couples today are childless and either the woman or the man, or possibly both, may be infertile. Infertility may result from a wide variety of causes. Some of the physical and hormonal causes may be

Special Needs

treatable, some not. If you are having trouble conceiving, you may even be told that there seems to be no reason why conception should not occur. Among animals, infertility and subfertility can be caused by faulty nutrition and it may be that in some cases of human infertility, a nutritional cause is partly or wholly responsible.

Miscarriage, stillbirth, handicap and low birth weight
The sperm or egg may be defective, or the embryo may be somehow abnormal and the woman may miscarry or a baby may develop which is not quite normal. Approximately one in five first pregnancies ends in a miscarriage. Even if the tiny embryo is perfectly formed some problem may occur later during pregnancy or at the birth. Around one in every ninety babies dies at birth or in the first few days of life. Only a tiny proportion of babies are handicapped but many more, approximately one in every thirteen, are born small (less than 5½ lb 2500 g). Small babies tend to have more health problems. Although faulty nutrition could be involved in some of these births, there are many other factors too which can affect the course and outcome of pregnancy.

If you do have, or have had, a miscarriage, stillbirth, handicapped baby or other problem during pregnancy, in some cases you may be told the possible reasons why. It could have been a physical problem such as cervical incompetence, an implantation in the wrong place, a serious medical condition, some problem which occurred during birth or a genetic defect.

Many handicaps are genetically determined, in other words, the infant inherits some defective genes from either or both of his parents. When prospective parents know of any defect which has appeared in more than one blood relative, it is wise to seek medical advice. If a longterm medical disorder was responsible for something going wrong during a previous pregnancy, it may be possible to be successful next time, with special medical care begun well before conception. The potentially harmful effects on a baby of genetic disorders, diseases or toxins have usually been considered to be entirely separate from other aspects of health such as what you eat and whether you smoke or drink etc. However, it is increasingly being realized that they are all inter-related and can influence each other. Whatever the cause, nutrition is still important.

As with infertility, in some cases something goes wrong even when there appears to be no reason, when to all intents and purposes both mother and father are healthy and have done all the 'right' things. It may be easier to understand how this could happen if you consider how complex the formation and transport of egg and sperm is, how quickly after fertilization the course of development takes place, and how complex the human baby is. Everything is working at top rate and there is no room for mistakes yet, just by the laws of chance, mistakes do occur sometimes.

If you do lose a baby or have a handicapped baby, it is very difficult to accept that the cause may be unknown. You may keep wondering why it should have happened to you and what you could possibly have done to cause it. If you have miscarried, it is little consolation to know that it is very common but this does mean that most of us probably know someone who has had a miscarriage. It can help to share your experiences with someone who has suffered a similar loss.

What can be particularly disheartening is if well-meaning people treat the problem lightly, as so often happens if you lose a baby in early pregnancy. You may even be advised to get pregnant again quickly, as if a baby were some easily replaceable commodity, when what you need is time – time to mourn the loss of your baby and time to recover your mental and physical health. The length of time will depend on a variety of things – how many months pregnant you were when you lost the baby, how well you are now and all the other circumstances of your life. Even after an early miscarriage (before twelve weeks), it is a good idea to leave three months, and longer if you can, before trying again. After a stillbirth or other loss in late pregnancy, it is worth considering leaving nine to twelve months before attempting to conceive, which will allow your body to recover fully and build up your nutritional reserves. This is a similar length of time to that you would leave if you had had a normal full term pregnancy.

Special Needs

What can you do?

You can do nothing about many of the factors which might affect whether you can conceive and what happens during pregnancy – your genetic constitution, your anatomy, past events during your own early development, even the compatibility or lack of it between the cells of you and your partner. Therefore it makes sense for both of you to concentrate on those aspects of your life which you are in control of and which could influence the course of pregnancy. This means being the right weight for your height, eating a well-balanced diet from all four food groups, with particular emphasis on foods which are rich sources of vitamins and minerals (see Chapter 9), and nourishing yourself generally (see Chapter 5).

Anaemia in pregnancy

This word is of Greek derivation meaning 'want of blood'. Certain anaemias can be inherited, for example, thalassaemia, and sickle cell anaemia. These are abnormalities of the haemoglobin in the blood. Women coming from countries where these disorders are common, such as Africa, the West Indies, Mediterranean countries and Asia, have a special blood test at their first ante-natal. But most anaemias are related to nutrition and are caused by a shortage of one or more of the many nutrients necessary for making haemoglobin in blood. In pregnancy, iron and folate deficiency anaemias commonly occur. Symptoms of anaemia may include pallor, lack of appetite, fatigue and lassitude. Blood tests during pregnancy assess your haemoglobin status, although changes in your body during pregnancy (such as the extra volume of blood) can make it difficult to diagnose iron deficiency accurately. This is why it is a good idea to have your iron status checked before as well as during pregnancy, especially if you have any of the symptoms described above and/or regularly lose large amounts of blood at menstruation.

As mentioned in Chapter 9, there is an increasing trend away from prescribing extra iron for all pregnant women; instead it is recommended that extra iron be given only to those whose blood tests show they are iron deficient after correcting for the physiological changes of pregnancy. Prevention of anaemia entails eating sufficient iron and folate-rich foods (see Chapter 9). Eating liver once a week and plenty of dark green vegetables will go a long way towards this.

Oedema, hypertension and pre-eclampsia

Oedema (swelling) can affect up to four out of five pregnant women and when it develops gradually and mostly affects the lower parts of the body, it is not necessarily a sign of anything wrong. It can cause concern when the oedema is generalized over the body and is linked with a sudden increase in weight, as this could indicate a potentially dangerous medical condition known as pre-eclamptic toxaemia (PET) or, more correctly, pre-eclampsia.

Hypertension (high blood pressure) can also be symptomatic of PET but again, not all women with high blood pressure will get PET. Some women have high blood pressure in pregnancy because they always have high blood pressure, others have a blood pressure which rises fairly suddenly during pregnancy. These women are monitored much more closely than usual. One reason why visits to the clinic become more frequent in later pregnancy is to keep a check on your blood pressure as well as to monitor your baby's continued wellbeing.

Who is most likely to suffer from PET? The commonly held view that it occurs more often in overweight women has not been well substantiated. If anything, it is the lighter than average woman who is more at risk. The number of theories as to what causes PET is almost as great as the number of remedies which have been tried. There is a higher incidence of PET in malnourished societies and good food and enough of it is the best way to guard against it. The latter part of pregnancy is not a time to eat less, especially if you have had PET in the past. If big meals are not appealing then eat smaller meals but eat more often so you are sure to be eating enough.

In Canada and the USA pregnant women who have had PET in a previous pregnancy are recommended, by some

Special Needs

nutritionists and doctors, to take extra calories and protein, above and beyond the normal pregnancy diet. Other research has suggested that extra calcium may help. An extra glass of milk and another egg a day above the basic pregnancy diet could make the difference. If you begin to show any signs or symptoms which might lead to PET, see your doctor without delay, eat more good food not less, and salt your food to taste. Salt-restricted diets and diuretics were popular at one time for treating PET but are now known to be ineffective and indeed may be dangerous for the pregnant woman.

If you have had PET in the past or wish to receive further information about this disorder, the organisation the Pre-eclamptic Toxaemia Society (PETS) publishes its own newsletter, can recommend a reading list and has a book-lending service (see address list on page 149).

EIGHT

Happy Birthday – and Afterwards

In between frequent visits to the antenatal clinic, you attend relaxation classes, pore over lists of items necessary for after the birth and trail round the shops seeking some elusive item of babygear. Or do you? Perhaps you are an old hand and still too busy feeding the rest of the family or wondering if you could just finish painting that skirting board before you are once again on 24-hour call.

The last few weeks of pregnancy

It becomes easy in the circumstances described above to neglect to eat properly. Nourishment is important through every stage of pregnancy and no less so in the last few weeks, when the baby is gaining a lot of weight and when brain growth and development is proceeding apace. At this stage a lot of nutrients will be going to the baby and you need to keep up the supply in order to prevent your own reserves being depleted and your own health being undermined. If you can't face large meals or feel too tired in the evening to prepare a meal, adapt to your changed circumstances. Eat simply prepared meals. Use some from the freezer, if you have one, and have put them away beforehand. Prepare snacks early in the day for consumption later when you are tired. Eat a good lunch rather than waiting to eat a big meal in the evening. Get someone else to do the heavy food shopping.

If a hospital birth is planned and you have a list of items to take, make a note of three extras to include – a small, real sponge (the expensive ragged-looking ones which can be obtained from chemists); some food for after the birth; and a packet of bran. Tips like these and those which follow are limited to the practical aspects of childbirth which relate to nutrition. It is not within the scope of this book to consider the deeply emotional aspects which are covered in detail elsewhere.

Happy Birthday – and Afterwards

Labour

For the very few, labour is a short event and there is no time to eat. For most of us it takes hours rather than minutes and nourishment is essential to prevent exhaustion.

The first stage of labour is usually characterized by regular but fairly weak contractions (similar to those you have been experiencing in the last few weeks). When this begins, if it is in the middle of the night, make yourself a hot drink then go back to bed and try to sleep or at least rest. You need to conserve your energy for later. If labour starts during the day, potter around doing what jobs you can comfortably manage and eat as normal.

When the contractions become stronger and longer (forty-five seconds to a minute) and you decide to prepare to leave for the hospital or phone the midwife, have something to eat (unless you have only just had a meal). This will be your last opportunity because later your digestive system slows down and you will be sick if you try to eat. Eating at this stage of contractions will enable your liver to restock its energy stores so that you can draw on them in the next few hours without becoming over-exhausted. Choose whatever you feel you can cope with: boiled egg and toast; a sandwich; some soup you may have already made; a milky drink; or maybe just a banana. Whoever prepares this meal should also check that you have some provisions in your bag for yourself after the birth, and for your birth attendant if someone is to accompany you. This will stand him or her in good stead if there is a long wait and there are no refreshment facilities open at the hospital.

In the second stage of labour, food and drink is the last thing you need but your mouth can become incredibly dry. Ask your companion to soak the small sponge in drinking water and squeeze it out lightly so that it is not dripping wet. Sucking and licking this between contractions can be unbelievably refreshing. (Do not use the sponge for everyday washing or anything else beforehand; soap-tainted water is not at all palatable). If labour goes on for a very long time and you feel exhausted, ask the midwife if you can have something

Eating Well for a Healthy Pregnancy

to restore your energy – perhaps a sweet drink or some glucose sweets. However, some labour wards do not permit these just in case you may need an anaesthetic, so it may be worth checking in advance with the hospital about their policy on food in labour.

After the birth

Your first drink may cause you to be sick, but it is of no significance when you have so much to think about and hopefully a baby to hold. It is a time for relief and happiness, tears of joy, or possibly of sadness.

Straight after the birth you certainly won't feel hungry, although after a while something sweet can be very restoring after the great physical effort of labour. A few hours later you will suddenly realize that you are not just hungry but absolutely ravenous. By some quirk of fate this often happens in the middle of the night or at some odd time during the day which seems hours away from the next scheduled meal. This is where your food provisions come in, and there's no doubt you've earned that first birthday meal.

After the birth your digestive system takes time to adjust. In the maternity ward there is great interest in your bowel movements; you'll soon know why, if you have stitches following the birth and become constipated. At the first opportunity after the birth when you can face it, with your first meal if possible, take a heaped teaspoon of the bran you brought (in milk, water or fruit juice or on cereal). Thereafter take 1 dessertspoon of bran every morning with your breakfast cereal until the danger period for constipation is over (usually just the first few days).

Often women who have had stitches 'hold back' for fear of doing some damage. If you have stitches, it is worth trying the following tip when you go to the toilet. Roll up a sanitary towel and sit forward on the seat so that the towel rests against the perineum (where the stitches are). Then you may feel more comfortable and able to function normally. Another thing which will help is to be mobile; so move around as soon as you are allowed to. Long spells immobile on the bed may make matters worse. Should it become necessary, there are laxative preparations which can relieve you without unduly upsetting the baby. If you are adamant about not taking anything by mouth, ask for a suppository instead.

The first few weeks of motherhood

Psychologically and physiologically you experience great changes after the birth. You may feel unusually high, you may be alternately elated and forlorn, or you may feel down in the depths for no apparent reason. It is wonderful to have a new baby but you also have to adapt to a non-stop daily routine, a lack of sleep which inexorably wears you down, and your own new feelings – not least of which may possibly be uncertainty over your ability to breast-feed or cope with the new responsibilities thrust upon you.

High on your list of priorities, place caring for your own diet – for your own sake, to aid recovery and minimize the chances of postnatal depression – and for the baby's sake, to ensure he or she gets an adequate supply of milk. Below is a summary check list of the four food groups for breast-feeding. Breastfeeding is the natural extension of pregnancy and childbirth. Your baby is outside the womb now but is normally still entirely dependent upon you for the next few months.

The four food groups for breast-feeding

The best diet for breast-feeding is one which supplies a little more of each nutrient than did your diet before or during pregnancy. You can eat a bit more of everything or increase the number of portions in the four food groups:

☐ *Meat and alternatives*
as in the diet recommended for pregnancy – see page 26 (chapter 2)
two large portions – four small or more.

☐ *Bread and cereals*
five to six portions (seven or more in a vegetarian menu)

☐ *Vegetables and fruit*
five (increase the portion size from that during pregnancy) or more than five portions (if you keep the portion size the same)

Eating Well for a Healthy Pregnancy

- ☐ *Milk and milk products*
  four to five portions
- ☐ *Fats and oils*
  extras taken after the food groups (1–2 tbsp)

Why breast milk is best

Breast milk is tailor-made for your baby. Artificial or 'formula' milks cannot compare. Despite the extremely hard work which manufacturers of baby milks have undertaken in the last few years to develop formulae as close as possible in composition to human milk, insurmountable differences still remain.

1. Human milk differs from other milks not only in its nutrients but also in 'biochemical' aspects. For example, your breast milk may contain substances which help to stimulate the digestive system of your newborn baby to develop.

2. Cows' milk has three times as much protein and more calcium in it than breast milk, because it is especially designed for a rapidly growing calf. The newer modified baby milks contain much less protein and calcium than cows' milk but some formula milks still differ quite a lot from human milk.

3. The baby's brain grows very rapidly in the months after the birth. The brain is largely lipid or fat and breast milk is rich in the special fats needed. Human milk is also very rich in lactose which supplies a substance called galactose needed too by the developing brain. Some of the formula milks contain less lactose than human milk.

4. Breast milk contains more cholesterol than cow's milk. Some people regard this as an important mechanism which allows the baby to adapt to coping with dietary cholesterol later in life.

5. Breast milk forms soft curds in the baby's stomach and the baby's motions or stools are mustard yellow and like thick custard – this is more natural for the baby; cow's milk formulae form tough rubbery curds in the baby's stomach and the motions are pale, bulky and firm.

6. Breast milk is ready mixed at the right dilution. If artificial milks are not made up correctly, the baby's fluid and mineral balance can be disturbed. Breast milk is also at the right temperature and requires no mixing.

7. Breast milk is a living fluid (it has been called 'white blood'), which contains enzymes (special proteins), hormones, and living cells. It is designed not only to feed your baby but also to guard against infection. The cells act as vigilantes warding off infection and gobbling up invaders. Human milk also contains a special substance called the bifidus factor, which encourages the growth of friendly organisms in the baby's intestines and these in turn help to deal with unwanted intruders. Artificial milk is 'dead' and cannot fulfil these functions so that the bottle-fed baby is more susceptible to tummy bugs and infections causing diarrhoea.

8. Breast milk is individually tailored for your baby. Cows' milk proteins are foreign and for some babies may be more likely to cause allergy if introduced too soon.

9. Breast-feeding encourages contraction of the uterus and helps the mother gradually to lose weight by drawing on the stores of fat which her body has laid down during pregnancy.

10. The baby's jaws work hard when breast-feeding and are stimulated to develop properly. Bottle feeding does not require the same effort.

11. Breast-feeding is economical. You may eat more but it need not be as expensive to do this as it is to buy artificial milks.

The possible disadvantages of breast-feeding
1. You are tied to the baby. However, even if it's not always easy, after the first weeks it is possible to arrange to be away for a feed on either a regular or occasional basis. Milk can be expressed manually or with a pump into a sterile container and stored a few hours or a day in the fridge, or longer in a freezer. If you yourself decide to try this and offer your own milk in a bottle, the baby might refuse because he senses your breast is there. Let someone else try – your baby may be more likely to accept a bottle from someone other than you.

2. You are the only one who can get up in the middle of the night. You can attempt to redress the balance after weaning.

3. Breast-feeding can for some be painful for the first few days. This wears off quite soon. The afterpains or contractions of the uterus when feeding in the early days are good for you but can be excruciating for several minutes at a time especially in mothers who have had another baby before. Make sure you are well supported by pillows before you start feeding, and have a warm water bottle for relief.

4. The baby may demand to be fed at frequent intervals and then go quite a long time before a subsequent feed. The pattern of bottle-fed babies is more regular.

5. Some people believe that breast-feeding spoils your breasts. This is a myth – the main enlargement of the breasts occurs during pregnancy and is unrelated to whether you breast-feed or not.

6. Human milk is low in iron. It does not make evolutionary sense for nature to make milk inadequate for its purpose and it has now been found that the baby can store iron for later use, in his or her own liver during the last few months of pregnancy; that 'late' clamping of the cord may benefit the baby's iron stores; and that the iron in human milk may be better absorbed than that in cow's milk-derived formulae. The presence of a larger amount of iron may not necessarily be beneficial as it may allow unwanted bacteria to flourish and may interfere with the baby's own anti-infective mechanisms.

7. There are certain rare circumstances in which breast milk may not be appropriate, for example, for the very premature baby and for certain medical conditions of either mother or baby. In all these cases, medical counselling and a full explanation of the reasons would normally be offered to the mother.

Making sure your breast milk is of the right quality
For the first few days after the birth you make colostrum, a yellowish viscous fluid. This protects the baby from infection, may have a laxative effect so helping to clear out

the meconium (the dark sticky first motions of your baby) and may also supply a concentrated dose of certain nutrients such as zinc.

A few days later, the colostrum is replaced by the thin bluish-white and very sweet breast milk. Providing you are well-nourished during pregnancy and continue to eat well whilst breast-feeding, you will produce milk which is the right quality for your baby, even though your milk differs from month to month, from week to week and even from hour to hour. It should not be necessary to take or give extra supplements.

If, conversely, your diet is inadequate in one or more nutrients, then your body stores may become depleted or the breast milk may reflect the deficiency. For example, if your diet were very low in vitamin C, so too would be your milk; if there were not enough calcium from your food for making milk, then calcium would be drawn from your bones. This may have undesirable effects on your long-term health and some nutritionists advise calcium supplements for women who normally have a very low intake of calcium for some special reason (such as inability to take dairy products).

One issue often raised when you begin breast-feeding is whether certain foods might affect the breast-milk and upset your baby. One well-meaning adviser may counsel you not to eat oranges or grapes, another may caution against cauliflower and cabbage, another may ban milk and another raw salads and spices. If you follow everyone's advice you may end up living on dry bread. While it is known that certain food constituents can pass into the milk, for example, from garlic, there is no evidence that these cause problems in the majority of babies, so eat what you fancy.

For a minority, foods such as chocolate may well provoke colic or vomiting in the baby and the only solution in such cases is trial and error. If problems recur frequently and you keep a diary of all foods and drinks taken in the four to six hours preceding that feed and a common item keeps cropping up, it may be worth excluding it for a day or two to see if you get any improvement. Remember though that babies do have an immature digestive system and colic can

Eating Well for a Healthy Pregnancy

occur without it being due to you. Of course the situation is quite different in those with allergic tendencies, and specialist advice may be necessary here.

The right quantity of breast milk

The aspect of breast-feeding which usually concerns mothers most is whether there is enough for the baby. If your baby has six or more wet nappies a day, is content between most (if not all) feeds and is gaining weight (after an initial loss), then he or she is having enough milk. Perhaps your baby is gaining well but is still discontented – try other ways of soothing such as cuddling or rocking. Maybe he or she just wants to be held or talked to. If your baby is not thriving, it is likely that you are failing to feed frequently enough or you are failing to let down the milk.

True physical inability to feed is very rare and it is unlikely that you would be unable to produce enough milk, *providing* the circumstances are right. This is the crux of the matter – all the surrounding circumstances need to be working together in your favour.

To breast-feed successfully, check the following:
1 Eat well

Women who are thin after the birth will need to eat a lot to satisfy their own and their baby's needs. Women who have the 'average' excess fat after the birth (9 lb or so), have 35,000 calories or 300 calories a day for the next three to four months from fat and will also need to eat more than usual to supply approximately another extra 500 calories daily. Some nutritionists stress that protein and energy (calories) are the most important needs, easily met by some extra milk every day. Others argue that the extra does not need to be rich in protein but can be met by a wide range of foods, for example taking just a little more of everything included in main meals or by an extra snack or two. Snacks are very helpful when breast-feeding but if you are busy it is all too easy just to grab some bread or a biscuit when it would be better eat a variety of snacks so that you gradually include something from all the different groups: fruit, nuts, cheese, milk, cold meat and raw vegetables as well as bread.

If you think your milk supply is inadequate, try eating a

Happy Birthday – and Afterwards

little extra in the form of several small meals a day. This is important particularly if you still have a lot of extra fat of your own. If you eat huge meals, the surplus to that immediately needed by you and the baby may go into your fat stores instead of into producing extra milk. Brewer's yeast gained a reputation in the past for increasing milk supply, but its efficacy has not really been proven.

2 *Drink enough*
Breast milk contains a lot of water. If your diet contains many foods in liquid form – milk, juices, soups – then a few extra glasses of water daily may be enough. Otherwise you may need six to ten drinks a day. You often feel thirsty when you feed the baby – get a drink ready before you begin or you may find yourself sitting feeling parched but reluctant to disturb the baby while you go and get a drink. Drinking more than you need will not increase supply. Do try to avoid vast quantities of tea or coffee as the baby may not be able to cope with caffeine as easily as you can.

3 *Feed your baby frequently*
This is especially important in the early weeks. A three- to four-hourly feeding regime might work for some but for others it could spell disaster. Frequent feeding is the norm in many societies and the composition of human milk is more similar to that of animals which feed more or less continuously than it is to animals which feed their young infrequently. You may find yourself feeding on average every two hours for several feeds and then have a long spell when no demand is made. Frequent feeding is also the best way for you to increase your supply. As the baby grows, his or her needs increase and on occasions may temporarily outstrip your supply. In this case, feed more often for a day or two until your body adapts to the new demands.

4 *Rest and relax*
Your home may be in chaos but try to put yourself and the baby first. When the baby sleeps, have a nap or at least a quiet time relaxing. If you are worn out, you may be more likely to be unable to let down the milk. Milk 'let down' is triggered by the physical stimulus of the baby sucking and by other stimuli such as the sight or sound of the baby or

Eating Well for a Healthy Pregnancy

even the thought of feeding. If you are relaxed, this will facilitate milk let down.

It is known that in many different societies, all manner of techniques, preparations and rituals were developed to stimulate milk flow. Nowadays, listening to music or reading a book whilst feeding can help you to relax. Privacy may be very important until you gain confidence. Drinking stout was often recommended in the past and certainly alcohol *in small amounts* may produce the necessary relaxation to allow milk let down. If you are having problems, it may be worth trying a small drink, possibly at the last feed in the evening. Larger quantities of alcohol may have the opposite effect and depress the let-down reflex as well as being potentially harmful to the baby. Anxiety or uncertainty can also block milk let down.

5 *Have a supporter*
If possible, have an attendant who can give information, physical help and emotional support while you are breast-feeding. This is an additional role of the midwife and it is also the purpose of the many breast-feeding support groups and counsellors (the Association of Breast-feeding Mothers, La Leche League and the National Childbirth Trust – see pages 147 and 149).

6 *Avoid things which might inhibit breast-feeding*
Try not to use oral contraceptives whilst breast-feeding because they can reduce the milk supply (but do use some form of contraception). Do *not* take other drugs until you have checked their safety with your doctor. Do not offer the baby supplementary or complementary feeds which will reduce rather than increase your supply. Leave the free milk samples and the promotional literature at the hospital or they might put you off breast-feeding.

A few thoughts on weaning

Weaning begins the first time you give your baby any nourishment other than milk. Introducing solids at too early an age may cause problems in some infants which could persist later in life, so as a general guideline it is now recommended that weaning be delayed preferably until around five to six months of age. There are exceptions to any rule; a big baby boy may be looking round for more before this age; conversely another baby may be quite content on milk alone for longer, although it has been suggested that the baby's needs for iron may not be fulfilled by milk alone after the first few months.

Be flexible. Don't have too many preconceived ideas about when you will wean and about what foods you will or will not give. A firm resolution to prepare absolutely everything yourself could prove impractical and frustrating on certain occasions. If you find yourself struggling with a sieve and spoon when you should have set off hours ago for a day out, it is worth considering a compromise. One way is to continue to prepare your own baby food most of the time but have some bought-in baby foods for emergency use, for introducing items you cannot easily make yourself and as reserves for when your own meal cannot be easily puréed.

Ideally, by the age of one year, your child will be eating a wide range of foods and sharing most meals with the rest of the family. So how does your baby progress from breast milk to the four food group infant diet? Fashions change in the order in which foods should be introduced. It is now recommended that cereals and cow milk are not introduced too early (before six months) to guard against the possibility of allergy. The baby's immature digestive system may not be able to cope with some of the proteins in these foods, or possibly with constituents of other foods such as egg. Your best guide on this is your baby – at first introduce foods one at a time in very small quantities and see what happens, both in your baby's reactions and the nappies.

If a food is not liked or seems to disagree, do not immediately assume that your baby is allergic (unless allergy runs in the family). True allergy is not very common and it does need expert diagnosis. If your baby is not really allergic to a food but just too young for it at present, it would be wrong to deprive him or her of this food for evermore. Try offering the food again in a small amount at some future date. On the other hand, if it *is* likely that your baby may have an allergic tendency, great care should be taken in these early months. Specialist advice may be needed and practical tips can be obtained from books and support groups. Prepared baby foods may contain a range of foods so that if, for example, you need to avoid milk, check that any packeted or tinned baby foods do not contain dried milk.

Some examples of foods to purée, sieve and offer in the latter half of the first year are shown below, in the different food groups.

☐ *Meat and alternatives*
Strained meat or the thick 'custard' which forms when blood runs out of meat and sets; white fish; egg yolk (only a very little at first); sieved pulses.

☐ *Bread and cereals*
Sieved porridge; baby muesli; bread (do not offer bread of too rough a texture at first. If you make your own, sieve the wholemeal flour finely and make special baby bread with little or no salt. You can slice and freeze this, then thaw one slice at a time. When signs of teething begin, hard crusts, baked slowly in the oven, can be offered); baby cereals (to avoid excessive weight gain, do not serve these too often); ground rice, semolina.
Delay all cereals where there is a tendency to allergy.

☐ *Vegetables and fruit*
Apple sauce, pears, apricots, peaches, ripe bananas, prunes.
Potato, peas, carrots, beetroot, marrow
(later) cabbage, Brussels sprouts, tomatoes.

☐ *Milk and milk products*
Whole milk (not skimmed, as it has been found to be undesirable for babies), cottage cheese, yogurt, cheese.
(Again delay if any allergic tendency)

Take weaning very gradually. Your baby's mouth has to cope with all kinds of different tastes and textures and with learning how to chew rather than suck. The rest of the digestive system has to adapt to new foods too. Very small quantities are recommended at first – $1/2$ to 1 teaspoon – and gradually these can be built up to tablespoon amounts. Similarly, progress from sterile (boiled) strained liquids (apple juice, carrot juice, meat juice) to a bit of solid pushed through the sieve to produce a fine-textured purée. This becomes less important later and mashing with a fork can gradually take over.

Be especially hygiene conscious and make sure that all utensils, bowls, sieves, mills or blenders are scrupulously clean. If you have a freezer, you can prepare foods in amounts sufficient for a few meals (e.g. puréed carrot, apple sauce, bone marrow broth) and spoon this into an ice-cube tray. After freezing, remove the cubes, bag, and keep in the freezer for a few weeks – the frozen food compartment of an ordinary fridge is not considered cold enough to inhibit bacterial growth completely. For a single baby meal, thaw one or more cubes as required and warm up. Do not refreeze any leftovers but discard them or eat them yourself. Whether you have a freezer or not, small quantities of the foods you are having yourself can be sieved at table (provided you add no salt during or after cooking).

Do not try to force your baby to eat, or push one spoonful of food in before the first has been savoured and swallowed. Let someone else spoonfeed you and you will quickly understand how the baby feels. As soon as your child can manage to feed him- or herself, whether it be with fingers or spoon, allow this. Some babies stubbornly refuse to be fed but will eat willingly, if messily, by themselves.

Eating with you, eating your foods and sharing his or her foods with you are part of the development of your baby's eating habits. Why should baby food be other than ordinary food except for its finer texture and lack of salt or other strong seasonings? If you rely completely on separate 'baby food' and separate baby meal times, you may pose yourself the eventual problem of weaning your child off 'baby' food on to 'real' food.

Your own nutritional needs Even when your baby has progressed on to the food enjoyed by the rest of the family, your day will still be full, the meticulous sieving and mashing being superseded by keeping track of a highly mobile and potentially destructive infant. You may not be as hungry as you were when fully breast-feeding but your needs will in all likelihood exceed those of before pregnancy because you will be more physically active now. Continue to keep foods

Eating Well for a Healthy Pregnancy

and their preparation as simple as possible to leave yourself as much time as you can.

The growing child and food rejection

Around the age of one to one-and-a-half, your child may suddenly become difficult over food, eat much less and reject completely foods which were previously acceptable. Maternal anxiety only seems to encourage the child's determination to resist. Make an objective assessment of the situation: does your child look well; is he or she about the right size and weight for age and lively during waking hours? It may seem to you that the baby is existing more or less on fresh air but what has happened is that food intake has slowed down because the rate of growth has slowed down. If your child doubled in weight every six months (as happened in the first six months), he or she would be enormous after a year or two! Concern is not necessary unless there is a real problem of failure to thrive, when you should seek help from the baby clinic.

Don't fall into the trap of fearing starvation and starting to offer biscuits and other between-meal snacks. Many children delight in existing on biscuits, much to the frustration of anxious parents. If one meal is refused, wait till the next – preferably, take your child away from food and kitchens and if possible outside for an appetite-raising session of exercise and fresh air.

At the next meal put on offer in the centre of the table not one food but a selection of single foods, which you are intending to have. (Some children at this age do not like mixed-up foods like stews, quiches etc). Sit down together and begin your meal. If your baby indicates a desire to eat and chooses one or more foods, serve only a small portion at first. Do not push any food; let him or her indicate what is wanted. Even the slightest degree of concern can be almost magically detected and seen as yet another opportunity to assert independence. Be aware of this even if you find it very difficult to remain entirely cool, calm and collected.

If all the foods on offer are refused, don't offer substitutes from cupboard or fridge and perform tricks to get the child to eat or you may be setting a precedent which you might regret. Accept your child's wishes and possible lack of hunger at that meal (don't rule out the possibility of tiredness; many very young children cannot eat when desperately in need of sleep). Wait until the next meal before offering alternatives. It is a good idea not to go to enormous lengths to prepare what you think are interesting dishes or your sense of frustration when he refuses to eat could be directly related to the length of time it took to prepare. Join a friend and her baby for lunch; it is easier to be calm about someone else's baby, as well as your own, not eating.

A child's inborn food sense
In conclusion, a tale, and possibly a lesson for us all. Many years ago an attempt was made to determine whether babies had any inborn food 'sense'. Babies of eight to nine months who had been fully breastfed up to that time, were allowed to choose by themselves what to eat and drink from a whole range of simple but wholesome foods: three meats (beef, lamb, chicken); four offal or organ meats (liver, brains, kidney, sweetbreads); yellow animal fat (bone marrow); seafish (haddock); full fat yogurt, whole milk; cereals (wholegrains); nine fresh vegetables (in season); five fresh fruits (again seasonal), and salt (served by itself not on or in any foods).

Somewhat to the surprise of the observers, the children took much more fruit, meat, eggs and fat than was – and still is – generally considered good for them. They took very much less of cereals and green leafy vegetables which were often popular with parents and some nutritionists. One child ate several eggs at one meal; another a huge portion of lamb; one had a 'jag' on beetroot; another touched no green leaves for six months or more. As they grew older, they did begin to eat more cereals and vegetables but not during the early months of the experiment.

No pressure to eat was ever exerted but just three meals a day were served with only water between meals. All the children tucked in at every meal; they grew well and were full of vigorous good health. Everything they ate agreed with them, not one was constipated, there were no cases of anorexia and in five years not one had stomach-ache. There were however enormous differences between individual children in the choice of foods but when their food intake over the course of a week was assessed scientifically, it was seen that the intake of protein, carbohydrate and fat bore an orderly relationship to each other, and to the children's requirements.

The conclusion of this study was that babies *do* have an innate ability to meet their own nutritional needs after weaning without detailed direction from parents *providing* that simple, fresh, unsophisticated and wholesome foods are on offer in abundance and that highly processed foods and drinks (cakes, biscuits, soft drinks) are not available. In other words, this is just the same kind of diet which the healthy societies described in Chapter 2 of this book were found to be taking.

NINE
Vitamins and Minerals

The importance of vitamins and minerals for a healthy pregnancy has been touched on many times already but this chapter, placed last because it is a little more technical than the rest of the book, is intended for those who have more than a passing interest in these nutrients.

Often people think of vitamins and minerals as substances which are somehow 'extra'. Yet it is worth noting that vitamins and minerals are, or should be, integral parts of the foods you eat every day. Supplementing the diet with added vitamins is a twentieth-century phenomenon; the word 'vitamin' was only invented in 1912. Bottled versions of these nutrients should not really be necessary, provided you eat a varied, well-balanced diet of mainly unrefined and fresh food. Then your intake of vitamins and minerals should be adequate for health and for pregnancy. But one of the main reasons why vitamins and minerals are so often the focus of attention nowadays is because many people today don't eat this kind of healthy diet. Instead we are increasingly faced with the problem of 'malnutrition of affluence' – ill-health caused by the long-term consumption of an imbalanced diet of highly refined and processed foods.

Why vitamins and minerals are so important to pregnancy

The widely known vitamins and minerals, with their common names and/or abbreviations are listed in the table on page 126. These play an integral part in the functions of the body and so are essential for good health and especially for pregnancy. If animals are fed a diet which contains enough of the major nutrients, protein, carbohydrate and fat, but which is severely deficient in one or more of the vitamins or minerals, then both male and female may become infertile.

VITAMINS

Abbreviation	Name (alternatives)
	Fat-soluble vitamins
A	Vitamin A (retinol)
proA	Carotene (provitamin A, a precursor of vitamin A)
D	Vitamin D (calciferol)
E	Vitamin E (tocopherol)
K	Vitamin K
	Water-soluble vitamins
B_1	Vitamin B_1 (thiamin)
B_2	Vitamin B_2 (riboflavin)
B_3	Niacin (nicotinic acid, nicotinamide)
B_6	Vitamin B_6 (pyridoxine)
B_{12}	Vitamin B_{12} (cobalamin)
B_c	Folic acid (folate, folacin)
	Pantothenic acid (pantothenate)
	Biotin
C	Vitamin C (ascorbic acid)

MINERALS

Abbreviation	Name
	Gross minerals (eaten in amounts of 100 mg or more daily)
Ca	Calcium
P	Phosphorus
Mg	Magnesium
Na	Sodium
K	Potassium
Cl	Chloride
	Trace elements (eaten in smaller quantities but still essential)
Fe	Iron
Zn	Zinc
Cu	Copper
Mn	Manganese
I	Iodine
F	Fluoride
Cr	Chromium
S	Sulphur
Se	Selenium
Mo	Molybdenum

Vitamins and Minerals

In one experiment in which groups of female rats were fed a diet lacking in just one vitamin for thirty-five days before mating, not a single rat succeeded in becoming pregnant. Even deficiencies which are less severe or not as prolonged and which do not seem to affect the general health or appearance of the mother, can still reduce fertility or cause death, malformation or growth retardation in the offspring. In the above experiment, other groups of rats were left without one vitamin for just thirteen days before mating. Far fewer rats conceived than would normally be expected to and those which did become pregnant and continued to eat the deficient diet were more likely to have smaller than average offspring, or babies which died or had handicaps.

It takes a special experiment to produce a diet *completely without* one or more of these essential nutrients and this could not happen with ordinary foods. However, although human diets may not be *completely* lacking in any one vitamin or mineral, it is now known that many women may be taking less than optimal amounts of these essential substances before as well as during pregnancy. Television advertisements, tempting displays of highly processed convenience foods, the ease of opening a packet or tin, together with a shortage of time, a lack of emphasis on the importance of nutritional education, and obsessions about dieting, can all combine to undermine the quality of what some people eat.

A professor in Leeds and another in South Wales have done some research so interesting to women that they are often quoted in women's and parents' magazines. In one study, women who had already had one or more babies with a special kind of handicap called a neural tube defect (for example, spina bifida or anencephaly) were prescribed a vitamin/mineral supplement by the doctor. They took this for at least four weeks before pregnancy and for the first eight weeks of pregnancy. These women were found to be seven times less likely to have another handicapped baby than similar women who did not take the supplement.

In the other study, similar women were given dietary advice and/or a supplement before as well as during early pregnancy. All the recurrences of handicap and nearly all

Eating Well for a Healthy Pregnancy

the miscarriages occurred in those women who, despite the advice given, failed to eat a good diet.

It is difficult to conduct research which measures vitamins and minerals in the diet, and any changes in these. A medical experiment with supplements can help to highlight how important some of the constituents of food are.

These studies together with other evidence have opened up the exciting prospect that not only spina bifida but other handicaps and problems of pregnancy may be preventable by paying more attention to food and to health before as well as during pregnancy. Sadly, the emphasis on good food as the best preparation for pregnancy has been neglected in some quarters; instead controversy has raged over the pros and cons of vitamin and mineral supplements.

Some people are strongly in favour of supplements being taken by every woman planning a pregnancy. This is largely because it can be very difficult to change people's long-entrenched eating habits, whereas it is a relatively easy matter to recommend taking a pill. However, many individuals are emphatically against this, their argument being that we do not yet know whether there could be risks associated with the longterm consumption of vitamin and mineral supplements, especially those containing rather high doses of certain ingredients.

Little publicity is given to the hazards of over-consumption of vitamins and minerals, yet excesses of certain of these nutrients can be just as damaging as deficiencies. Such excesses cannot be achieved by food alone, unless some very weird and bizarre diet is eaten. Yet it is possible to overdose oneself with some of the supplements which are available, although the majority contain vitamins and minerals in amounts that you might obtain from food sources.

The most well-known examples of vitamin toxicity are the fat-soluble vitamins A and D. These can accumulate in the body and excess can definitely harm both mother and baby. Vitamins E and K are also fat-soluble but far less toxic. The other major group of vitamins are the water-soluble which include the B complex and vitamin C. These have traditionally been considered to be quite safe, since

Vitamins and Minerals

any excess would leave the body in the urine, but now that the fashion for taking 'megadoses' (amounts greatly exceeding what you would normally get from food, e.g. 1 g or 1000 mg of vitamin C compared to the 100 mg or so obtainable daily from food) is growing, so too is the evidence that such megadoses, especially if taken long-term, may not always be beneficial.

Many of us appreciate how large doses of vitamin C (1 g or 1000 mg or more daily) can help to treat the common cold. However, taking such doses all the time, especially before and during pregnancy, may not be such a good idea. A few isolated reports have suggested that such an excess of vitamin C may make it more difficult for a woman to conceive, that women who do take megadoses in very early pregnancy may be slightly more at risk of miscarriage, and that taking large doses for a long time may cause dependency so that suddenly stopping might lead to symptoms of vitamin C deficiency. With this in mind, if you do decide to take any supplementary vitamin C, it may be worth considering limiting it to no more than 100-200 mg per day (or best of all concentrating on good food sources of this vitamin) and before you take any supplement discuss it with your doctor.

No less interesting is the debate over a mineral – iron – in pregnancy. It may not really be necessary to have to suffer the constipation, diarrhoea or other side effects of that daily iron pill whilst you are pregnant. Recent studies have shown that women *who do not need extra iron* may not derive any benefit from taking a lot of extra iron. It is a different matter if blood tests have shown a deficiency of iron. Then a supplement may be needed – and/or lots of good food sources of readily absorbable iron such as that present in meat and liver. Just to complicate matters further, suppose that a woman who does need iron is also low on zinc. Giving her massive doses of iron in a supplement might lead to a zinc deficiency, because of the complex and delicate interactions between minerals. Yet food sources of iron can also be good sources of zinc. Zinc is another mineral needed for healthy reproduction.

All this may seem very complicated, and it is. The interactions between minerals and other minerals, between vitamins and other vitamins, and between vitamins and minerals, *are* incredibly complex. For the majority of women, the self-help way to obtain vitamins and minerals is from good food. For some women, supplements may be recommended and those which contain a wide range of vitamins and minerals in reasonable amounts may be best. If you are advised by your doctor to take such supplements, do so. However, the scientists probably still don't know all there is to know about vitamins and minerals and their interactions, so do not assume that bad food plus a vitamin/mineral supplement equals good food. A vitamin and mineral supplement may be helpful but if you do have to take one, eat the best diet you can as well.

How to assess whether you need extra vitamins and minerals

A vitamin/mineral deficiency may take a very long time to develop and it can be caused by several things, of which poor food or poor choice of food, is the main one. This and other causes are shown in the diagram on the opposite page, which also illustrates the various stages in the development of a deficiency and at which stages the deficiency might be detectable.

If your doctor thinks an assessment of your vitamin and mineral status is necessary, he may use one or a combination of different methods, which might include:

dietary analysis, which assesses the general quality of your diet and could also be used to estimate the approximate amounts of vitamins and minerals you eat,

laboratory tests which measure the levels of vitamins or minerals in various body tissues, such as blood, urine, hair and saliva,

clinical assessment, which concentrates on the careful observation of certain areas of the body, such as eyes, mouth and skin.

Before pregnancy, although the services of an NHS dietitian are available in most parts of the country, referral is usually only via a doctor. Many dietitians have a very heavy

Vitamins and Minerals

Development of a Vitamin/Mineral Deficiency, and Recovery

Change in diet or health — *Consequences*

{
POOR DIET
(poor quality food, wrong choice of food, not enough to eat)
Detectable by dietary analysis

EXTRA NEEDS
(growth, pregnancy)

MEDICAL DISORDERS
(malabsorption)

INFECTION
}

→ **SUPPLY FAILS TO MEET DEMAND**
Body uses vitamins and minerals, stores begin to be used

↓

STORES BEGIN TO FALL
No obvious signs
Lab tests may be normal

↓

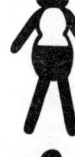

STORES DROP FURTHER
Still no outward signs
May be detectable by lab tests
Baby may be at risk

↓

STORES EVEN LOWER
Mother may be unable to conceive
If conceives, baby at risk

↓

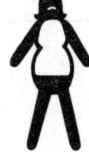

BODY STORES ALMOST DEPLETED
Usually outward signs e.g. in skin, mouth, tongue
Detectable by clinical observation
Usually infertile

↓

{
CHANGE TO GOOD DIET
(possibly supplementation)

INFECTION OVER

MEDICAL DISORDER

RECEIVES ATTENTION
}

→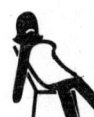

BODY STORES BEGIN TO REPLENISH
Mother takes precedence
Baby may still be at risk

↓

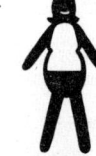

BODY STORES NORMAL
Full health and vitality
Vitamins and minerals available for mother and baby

AT RISK ZONE FOR PREGNANCY

workload and may only be able to see special cases. (Information about dietitians working privately may sometimes be available from your doctor or from an advertisement in your local newspaper by the dietitian involved. Always check out the qualifications of a dietitian before following his/her advice.) During pregnancy, the dietitians who work in the ante-natal clinic offer guidelines on general good nutrition; on rare occasions a detailed assessment of vitamin and mineral intake may be made.

Some modern laboratory tests for measuring vitamins and minerals in blood, urine and saliva, may be able to detect deficiencies before they begin to have a marked effect on your general health and well-being. These tests may have disadvantages – sometimes accurate interpretation of results may be difficult and a single sample may not be a reliable indicator of normal levels. This is because the concentrations of some nutrients in different tissues can fluctuate a great deal, depending on such things as the time of the last meal, the time of day, month or even the season of the year. This helps to explain why sometimes more than one test may be needed or why you may be asked to come at a particular time of day and perhaps be asked not to eat beforehand.

Hair analysis is a technique for assessing the levels of minerals in hair but this is not currently available through the NHS. A veritable hair analysis industry has mushroomed into being in the United States and looks like following suit in the UK. However, a few words of caution may be useful before you rush for the scissors and cheque book. In the future, hair analysis may be of great benefit for the diagnosis of an individual's mineral status but many eminent scientists have stated that this is not yet feasible and will not be until a lot more research has been completed.

Certainly the technique is worthless for vitamins, and the problems of mineral analysis centre on the overwhelming difficulties involved in the interpretation of hair charts. Many things can affect the levels of minerals in the hair – the external environment, washing procedures, hair treatments such as dyes, perms and even shampoos which contain minerals such as selenium or zinc, the natural colour of hair, the person's age and sex, the season of the year and the rate of hair growth. The levels of minerals in the hair do not often correspond to the levels in blood, urine or saliva, which makes it even more difficult to relate the values to your own health. One area in which hair analysis *may* prove useful is in the detection of high levels of toxic minerals such as lead, mercury and cadmium. A high result here would be well worth following up with further tests of blood and urine.

In the clinical assessment of a vitamin/mineral deficiency, the doctor concentrates on external signs and symptoms. These are usually only apparent when the deficiency has become severe, and has been caused by long periods on an inadequate diet or by certain medical conditions. Some examples of the signs symptomatic of specific vitamin deficiencies are:

- The scurvy and bleeding gums of vitamin C deficiency.
- The 'beefy' tongue and dermatitis on the exposed skin of neck, hands and feet of niacin deficiency.
- The deeply fissured tongue and cracks at the side of the mouth of riboflavin deficiency.
- The poor dark adaptation or 'night blindness' of vitamin A deficiency.

Such symptoms rarely occur in this country but there are some more general signs and indicators given in the list below which can be attributable to poor nutrition or to undernutrition. There can, however, be other reasons for such symptoms – certain diseases or medical disorders – so if you suffer from any of the following, do consult your doctor:

- *General appearance*
  Listless, easily tired, no energy, lethargic
- *Skin*
  Rough, dry, scaly, pale, pigmented
- *Nails*
  Spoon-shaped, brittle, ridged, lots of white flecks

Eating Well for a Healthy Pregnancy

☐ *Mouth*
Swollen, cracks in corners; lips dry and scaly; tongue swollen, very red or fissured; gums spongy, inflamed or bleed easily.

☐ *Eyes*
Poor dark adaptation, feeling of grittiness, dryness of eyes

☐ *Digestive system*
Poor appetite, indigestion, constipation, diarrhoea

☐ *Nervous system*
Confusion, irritability, inattentiveness, psychoses

How to get extra vitamins and minerals

Eating good food, the right kinds of food and enough of it, is by far the best way to get the vitamins and minerals you need. Additional ways to obtain these nutrients include the traditional food 'extras' and the bottled or packaged supplements.

Food sources
One way to remember which foods are good sources of vitamins and minerals is to think of the foods which are purpose-made products for the development of a young animal or plant, such as milk and eggs, seeds such as wheat, oats, rice, beans and nuts, or those storage organs within the animal or plant, such as liver and carrots.

Vitamins and minerals are found in clusters in foods; so for example, when you eat an orange you get not only vitamin C but also the vitamin folate; eat a serving of Brussels sprouts and you consume a cocktail of vitamins and minerals.

The tables on pages 136–139 are a brief guide to some of the good sources of the various vitamins and some of the minerals. But even among foods which seem good sources of minerals there is great variation in how readily these minerals are absorbed by your body. For example, the calcium in milk is better absorbed than calcium from other sources; the iron in meat is better absorbed than that from vegetables.

Vitamins and Minerals

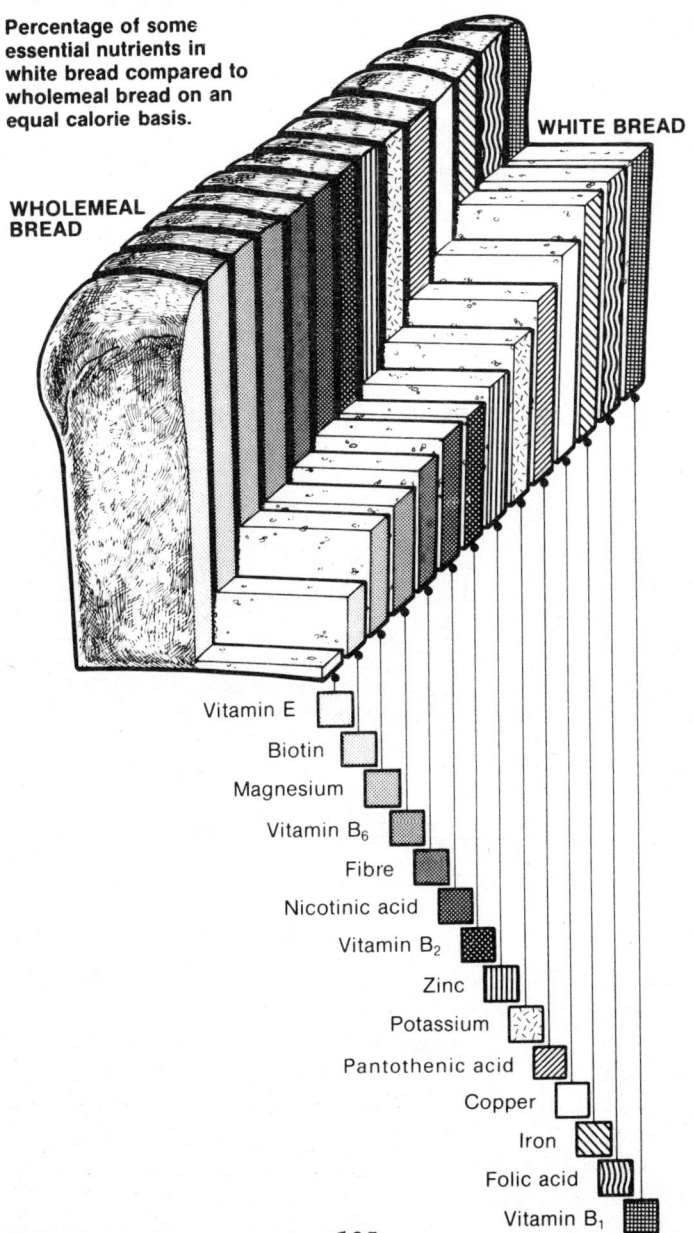

Percentage of some essential nutrients in white bread compared to wholemeal bread on an equal calorie basis.

WHOLEMEAL BREAD

WHITE BREAD

Vitamin E
Biotin
Magnesium
Vitamin B₆
Fibre
Nicotinic acid
Vitamin B₂
Zinc
Potassium
Pantothenic acid
Copper
Iron
Folic acid
Vitamin B₁

Guide to good sources of nutrients

Vitamins	Meat and alternatives	Bread and cereals	Milk and milk products	Fruit and vegetables	Other sources
A (carotene)	liver*, oily fish, eggs, kidneys		butter, cheese, milk	(carrots, green leafy vegetables, French beans, apricots, bananas, tomatoes)	fish liver oils*
D	eggs*, liver, oily fish		cream, butter, cheese		sunlight*, fish liver oils*
E	seed oils, egg yolk, peanuts, seeds	wheatgerm, wholegrain cereals	milk and milk products	vegetable oils, broccoli	yeast
K	lean meat, liver			broccoli, kale, spinach, tomatoes	made in gut by bacteria
B_1	seeds, nuts, peas, beans, pork, liver	brown rice, wholegrain cereals and bread, bran*			yeast*
B_2	eggs*, meat, kidney, fish	brown rice, wholemeal bread	milk, cheese	spinach, leafy vegetables	

Vitamins and Minerals

Niacin	meat*, fish*, beans, peas, nuts	wheat and wholewheat products		fruit and vegetables	yeast*
B₆	liver, beef, oily fish*, peas, beans	wholegrain products	Brie and Camembert cheeses	bananas, carrots, avocado, spinach	yeast*
B₁₂	kidney, liver, oxliver*, heart, eggs, herrings, mackerel		milk, cheese		
Folate	liver*, kidney*			spinach, dark green vegetables, oranges	yeast
Pantothenic acid	liver*, peas, kidney, eggyolk, seafish	wheatgerm	milk, cheese	mushrooms, spinach, potatoes	yeast*
Biotin	liver*, nuts, kidney*, lentils, eggs, meat and poultry	wholegrain cereals, wholemeal flour, brown rice	milk, cheese	cauliflower	yeast*
C				blackcurrants, grapefruit, lemons, oranges, strawberries, broccoli*, cauliflower, spinach*, cabbage* Brussels sprouts* (when fresh)	hips and haws

Eating Well for a Healthy Pregnancy

Minerals	Meat and alternatives	Bread and cereals	Milk and milk products	Fruit and vegetables	Other sources
Calcium	sardines, soya	wheatgerm	milk, cheese, yogurt	watercress**	yeast
Magnesium	meat, poultry, fish, seafood, nuts*, dried soyabeans, dried peas	wholemeal flour, brown rice, wholegrain cereals	milk	leafy green vegetables	brewer's yeast
Iron	beef, kidney*, liver*, eggs, sardines, haricot beans, lentils, almonds	wholemeal bread, oats, crispbread		potatoes, tomatoes, cabbage, broccoli, beetroot, dried apricots, figs, prunes**	yeast, cocoa, curry powder, ginger, mustard, blackstrap molasses
Zinc	beef*, liver*, seafood, oysters*, nuts, peanuts, peas	wholemeal bread	cheese	carrots, sweetcorn, tomatoes	yeast, ginger, mustard
Copper	calf liver*, lobster*, nuts, beans	wheatgerm		olives	yeast

Vitamins and Minerals

Chromium	liver	wheatgerm	cheese	brewer's yeast, black pepper, molasses, raw sugar
Manganese	hazelnuts*, peas, beans, coconut, almonds	wholemeal bread*, oatflakes*, wheatgerm, brown rice		leaves – spinach, watercress, avocado*, pineapple, plums	tea
Selenium	eggs, fish, meat, poultry, organ meats, nuts	wholegrain cereals			

* especially rich sources
** spinach, watercress, wheatgerm and lentils, although containing large amounts of iron (and other minerals) also contain substances which can inhibit the absorption of these minerals (see Chapter 7 page 98, on vegetarian/vegan diets).

Eating Well for a Healthy Pregnancy

Look at the tables and see if there is any food or foods which you might enjoy but have got out of the habit of eating or maybe which you have never even tried. Underline the things you seldom or never eat and begin to try them, one or two at a time. The fewer things you underline as seldom eaten, the better and more varied your diet.

Your intake of vitamins and minerals can vary a great deal depending not only on which foods you choose to eat but on the extent to which they have been refined and processed. The illustration on page 135 compares the relative proportions of vitamins, minerals and fibre in white versus wholemeal bread. If you refer back to the one day's eating plan in Chapter 2 (pages 28–29), it is easy to see which diet contains more vitamins and minerals. In Chapter 4 (pages 52–53), the shopping baskets for a family of four differed greatly in the relative proportions of vitamins and minerals as well as in those of major nutrients.

The degree of food refining and processing will affect the vitamin and mineral content but so too does the way in which foods are grown and the length of time in storage. New potatoes can contain up to five times as much vitamin C as old potatoes. Fresh leafy vegetables will lose vitamin C rapidly during storage, especially if they wilt. Cooking can cause further losses of vitamins and minerals though such losses can be minimized by careful cooking in a minimum of water as described earlier and by using the resultant stock in soups, sauces and gravies.

Food extras

Certain traditional food extras are naturally rich sources of some of the vitamins and minerals. Examples include:

☐ *Brewer's yeast*
  B vitamins (B_1, B_2, niacin, B_6, folate), vitamin E and the minerals iron, magnesium, copper, zinc and chromium.

☐ *Wheatgerm*
  B vitamins, vitamin E, and the minerals iron, calcium, magnesium, copper, zinc.

☐ *Codliver oil*
  Vitamins A, D and E and the essential fatty acids (you

Vitamins and Minerals

would need to consume a very large quantity for it to be toxic but it is advisable not to exceed the stated dose).

- ☐ *Kelp (seaweed)*
  Minerals.

- ☐ *Liver extracts*
  B vitamins and minerals.

- ☐ *Yeast extracts* (Bovril, Marmite etc)
  B vitamins.

Vitamin and mineral supplements
There may be special circumstances which make it necessary for you to take a supplement. For example, if you have a medical condition which affects your vitamin/mineral status or have to take drugs which increase the need for these nutrients; if you have experienced some problem in a previous pregnancy which might have been related to vitamins and minerals; or if, for any reason, you cannot eat the well-balanced diet described in this book.

It may be that your doctor will prescribe a supplement or you may decide to buy one of the multitude of supplements now available over the counter. Of those on sale, the supplements which contain a wide range of vitamins and minerals, in amounts which approximate to the quantities you might obtain from food, are usually the most suitable. Beware of elaborate packaging; this often means the supplement is much more expensive but not necessarily any better than those which are more simply packaged and less expensive.

Reading List

Below is just a small selection of follow-up reading. Within the confines of this book, it is impossible to cite all the books, research and review papers to which reference was made.

CHAPTER ONE: IT TAKES TWO

Carter, Margaret (ed), *0 to 5. The Complete Handbook for Young Mothers*. Grosvenor Press, 1983. (Contains a section for fathers.)

Elam, Daniel, *Building Better Babies. Preconception Planning for Healthier Children*. Celestial Arts, California, 1980. (Includes a chapter on sperm.)

Loader, Ann (ed), on behalf of The National Childbirth Trust, *Pregnancy and Parenthood*. Oxford University Press, 1982.

Phillips, Angela, *Your Body, Your Baby, Your Life*. Pandora Press, 1983.

Trimmer, Dr E. (ed.), *You're a Father*. Pagoda Books, 1983.

Wynn, Margaret and Arthur, *The Prevention of Handicap and the Health of Women*. Routledge and Kegan Paul, London, 1979.

Wynn, Margaret and Arthur, *The Prevention of Handicap of Early Pregnancy Origin*. Foundation for Education and Research in Childbearing, 27 Walpole Street, London SW3. (Technical.)

CHAPTER TWO: HEALTHY EATING

(General Nutrition)

Balfour, Lady Eve, *The Living Soil and the Haughley Experiment*. Universel Books, New York, 1975. (See Chapter 7, Whole Diets.)

Crawford, Michael and Sheilagh, *What We Eat Today*. Neville Spearman, London, 1972.

Reading List

Gear, Alan (ed), *The Organic Food Guide*. Henry Doubleday Research Association, 1983.

Grant, Doris, *Your Daily Food: Recipe for Survival*. Faber and Faber, 1973.

McCarrison, Sir Robert, *Nutrition and Health*. The McCarrison Society, 76 Harley Street, London, 1982.

Price, Dr Weston, *Nutrition and Physical Degeneration*. Price-Pottenger Foundation, New York, 1945, Heritage Edition, 1972. Obtainable from Wholefood (see address list, page 150).

(Nutrition and Pregnancy)

Cronin, Isaac, and Brewer, Gail S., *Eating for Two*. Bantam, New York, 1983.

Williams, Phyllis S., *Nourishing your Unborn Child*. Avon, New York, 1982.

Worthington-Roberts, Bonnie S., Vermeersch, J., and Rodwell-Williams, S., *Nutrition in Pregnancy and Lactation*. 2nd edn. C.V. Mosby Company, London, 1981. (Technical.)

CHAPTER THREE: DOES WEIGHT MATTER?

Cannon, Geoffrey, and Einzig, Hetty, *Dieting Makes You Fat*. Century Publishing, London, 1983.

Crisp, A. H., *Anorexia Nervosa: Let Me Be*. Academic Press, London, 1980.

Garrow, J.S., *Treat Obesity Seriously: a Clinical Manual*. Churchill Livingstone, Edinburgh, 1981. (Technical.)

Lambley, P., *How to Survive Anorexia: a Guide to Anorexia Nervosa and Bulimarexia*. Frederick Muller Ltd., London, 1983.

Macleod, Sheila, *The Art of Starvation*. Virago, 1981.

Orbach, Susie, *Fat is a Feminist Issue*. Hamlyn, 1978.

CHAPTER FOUR: PUTTING THEORY INTO PRACTICE

Davenport, Diana, *One Parent Families: a Practical Guide to Coping*. Sheldon Press, 1982.

Davis, Adelle, *Let's Cook it Right*. Unwin paperback, London, 1977.

Elliot, Rose, *The Bean Book*. Fontana, 1979.

Horley, Georgina, *Good Food on a Budget*. Penguin Handbook, 1972.

Jervis, Norman and Ruth, *The Foresight Wholefood Cookbook*. Roberts Publications, 1984.

Lewis, Catherine, *Good Food before Birth*. Unwin paperback, 1984.

Look at the Label. A booklet by the Ministry of Agriculture, Fisheries and Food, explaining what the labels on prepacked foods mean. Write to MAFF, Publications Unit, Lion House, Willowburn Trading Estate, Alnwick, Northumberland NE66 2PF.

Smith, Delia, *Frugal Food*. Coronet, 1976.

Trum Hunter, Beatrice, *The Natural Foods Cookbook*. Faber and Faber, London, 1975.

CHAPTER FIVE: NOURISHING YOURSELF AND YOUR BABY

Barlow, S.M. and Sullivan, F.M., *Reproductive Hazards of Industrial Chemicals*. Academic Press, 1982. (Technical.)

Durward, Lyn, and Evans, Ruth (eds.), *Maternity Rights Handbook* (see chapter on work hazards by Bronwen Bernard.) Penguin, 1984.

Guillebaud, John, *The Pill*. 2nd edn. Oxford University Press, 1983.

Madders, Jane, *Stress and Relaxation*. Martin Dunitz, London, 1979.

Mitchell, Laura, *Simple Relaxation*. John Murray, 1977.

Neumann, Dr H.H., *Dr. Neumann's Guide to the New Sexually Transmitted Diseases*. Acropolis, Washington, 1983.

Pelletier, K.R., *Mind as Healer, Mind as Slayer*. Dell Publishing Co. Inc., New York, 1977.

Sidle, Dr Nick, *Smoking and Pregnancy: a Review*. Hera Research Unit, The Spastics Society, 1982. (Technical.)

The National Council of Women Working Party on Alcohol Problems, *Alcohol and the Unborn Child*. 36 Lower Sloane Street, London SW1, 1980.

Reading List

Wynn, Margaret and Arthur, *Lead and Human Reproduction*. Evidence to the Royal Commission on Environmental Pollution. Clear Charitable Trust, 2 Northdown Street, London, 1982. (Technical.)

CHAPTER SEVEN: SPECIAL NEEDS

Baldwin, Dorothy, *Understanding Your Baby*. Ebury Press, 1983. (Particularly suitable for teenage mothers-to-be.)

Brewer, Gail, Sforza, *What Every Pregnant Woman Should Know*. Penguin, 1979. (About pre-eclampsia.)

Elliot, Rose, *Rose Elliot's Vegetarian Baby Book*. Fontana, 1984.

Friedrich, E. and Rowlands, P., *The Twins Handbook*. Robson Books, 1983.

Kitzinger, Sheila, *Birth Over Thirty*. Sheldon Press, 1982.

Minchin, Maureen, *Food for Thought: a Parent's Guide to Food Intolerance*. Allen and Unwin, Australia, 1983.

Moore Lappé, Frances, *Diet for a Small Planet*. Ballantine Books, New York, 1982. [See also the book listed for Chapter Two: *Eating for Two*, which has sections on vegetarian and vegan diets for pregnancy.]

Oakley, Ann, McPherson, Dr Ann, and Roberts, Helen, *Miscarriage*. Fontana, 1984.

CHAPTER EIGHT: HAPPY BIRTHDAY AND AFTERWARDS

Borg, Susan and Lasker, Judith, *When Pregnancy Fails*. Routledge and Kegan Paul, 1983.

Boyd, Catherine and Sellers, Lea, *The British Way of Birth*. Pan and The Spastics Society, 1982.

Caesarean Birth: a Handbook for Parents. Published by the Caesarean Support Group of Cambridge 1982. Available from Ann Watson, 7 Green Street, Willingham, Cambs. £1.50.

Guide to Breastfeeding. Booklet produced by the Bromley and District Branch of the National Childbirth Trust. Send 70p (Plus 25p p & p) to Anne Unseld, 42 Kent Road, West Wickham, Kent BR4 0JP.

Jelliffe, D.B. and Jelliffe, E.F. Patrice, *Human Milk in the Modern World*. Oxford University Press, 1978. (Technical.)

Kitzinger, Sheila, *The Experience of Childbirth*. Victor Gollancz Ltd., 1972.

Leboyer, Frederick, *Birth Without Violence*. Fontana, 1975.

Lewis, Catherine, *Growing Up with Good Food*. Unwin Paperbacks, in association with the National Childbirth Trust, 1982.

Messenger, Máire, *The Breastfeeding Book*. Century, 1982.

Odent, Michel, *Entering the World: The Demedicalisation of Childbirth*. Marion Boyars, 1983.

Stanway, Drs Penny and Andrew, *Breast is Best: a Commonsense Approach to Breastfeeding*. Pan, 1978.

Stanway, Drs Andrew and Penny, *Choices in Childbirth*. Pan, 1984.

Wright, Erna, *The New Childbirth*. Star (W.H. Allen & Co.), 1979.

CHAPTER NINE: VITAMINS AND MINERALS

Gildroy, Ann, *Vitamins and Your Health*. George Allen and Unwin, London, 1982.

Marks, John, *A Guide to the Vitamins*. MTP Press, Lancaster, 1983. (Technical.)

Mervyn, Len, *Minerals and Your Health*. George Allen and Unwin, London, 1980.

Underwood, E.J., *Trace Elements in Human and Animal Nutrition*. Academic Press, New York and London, 4th edition, 1977.

List of Useful Addresses

Please send a large, stamped addressed envelope with requests for information.

Action Against Allergy, 43 The Downs, London SW20 8HG (01-947 5082). An association to further the study of the role of modern foods, chemicals and biological materials in the cause of allergy.

Active Birth Movement, 32 Cholmeley Crescent, Highgate, London N6 5JR.

Anorexic Aid, The Priory Centre, 11 Priory Road, High Wycombe, Bucks. Send SAE for leaflet, information about local groups, and reading list. Also has information on other eating disorders e.g. bulimia and binge-eating.

Association For Breastfeeding Mothers. Peggy Thomas, 131 Mayow Road, London SE26. For telephone counselling 01-461 0022.

Association For Improvements In Maternity Services (AIMS). The Secretary: Christine Rogers, 163 Liverpool Road, London N1 0RF.

Association For Postnatal Illness, 7 Gowan Avenue, Fulham, London SW6.
Send SAE for leaflet. Also publishes a regular newsletter.

The Birth Centre, 101 Tufnell Park Road, London N7 0PE. (01-609 7466).
Publishes a quarterly newsletter, also leaflets, lists of local groups and teachers who advise on preparation for birth and yoga for pregnancy.

The British Diabetic Association, 10 Queen Anne Street, London W1M 0BD.
For further information on diabetes and pregnancy.

The British Goat Society. Angela Bell, P.R.O., Blacknest Lodge, Blacknest Road, Sunningdale, Ascot, Berks.
For addresses of local suppliers of goat milk.

Caesarean Support Group Of Cambridge. Katherine Steele, 7 Aylestone Road, Cambridge.

Eating Well for a Healthy Pregnancy

Campaign For Lead-Free Air (CLEAR), 2 Northdown Street, London N1 9BG.
Produces information and a newsletter. Welcomes help at national and local level.

Citizens' Advice Bureau, 31 Wellington Street, London (01-379 6841).
For information about local offices. No charge for counselling.

Council On Alcohol Related Problems, 12 Lombard Street, Belfast, BT1 1RD.
Send SAE plus 10p for leaflet on alcohol and pregnancy.

Depressives Associated, 19 Merley Ways, Wimborne Minster, Dorset BH21 1QN.

DHSS Leaflet Unit, PO Box 21, Stanmore HA7 1AY.

Disability Alliance, 25 Denmark Street, London WC2 8NJ.
For information on rights, benefits and services, for all people with disabilities, and their families.

Foodwatch, High Acre, East Stour, Gillingham, Dorset SP8 5JR.
A technical advisory service, particularly for people with needs for special foods.

Foresight: The Association For The Promotion of Preconceptual Care, The Old Vicarage, Church Lane, Witley, Godalming, Surrey, GU8 5PN. (042879 4500 from 9.30 – 7.30 p.m.).
Has a wide range of booklets on preconception care (e.g. *Guidelines for Future Parents* £1.20 plus SAE); also a newsletter and information about private preconception clinics, hair analysis and vitamin/mineral supplements.

Gingerbread, 35 Wellington St., London WC2 (01-240 0953).
For one parent families. Information sheets and register of local groups.

Health and Safety Executive, St Hugh's House, Trinity Rd., Bootle, Liverpool, L20 3QY (051-951 4000).
For information about work hazards.

Health Education Council, 78 New Oxford St., London WC1A 1AH.
For leaflets on general health, pregnancy, breast-feeding and giving up smoking.

Hyperactive Children's Support Group, Sally Bunday, 59 Meadowside, Angmering, West Sussex.

Henry Doubleday Research Association, Convent Lane, Bocking, Braintree, Essex CM7 6RW.
For information about organic farming and growing.

List of Useful Addresses

The Herpes Association, c/o Spare Rib Ltd, 27 Clerkenwell Close, London EC1.

La Leche League, Box BM 3424, London WC1V 6XX.
For information about breast-feeding, local support groups and counselling.

Maternity Alliance, 59-61 Camden High Street, London NW1 7JL (01-388 6337).
Publishes a regular bulletin 'Maternity Action' plus leaflets; 'Money for mothers and babies', 'Single payments for babygoods', 'Getting fit for pregnancy', 'Pregnant at work'. Send SAE for information on membership and/or leaflets.

Meet A Mum Association, 26a Cumnor Hill, Oxford OX2 9HA.

The Miscarriage Association, Dolphin Cottage, 4 Ashfield Terrace, Thorpe, nr Wakefield, Yorks.
For information on local groups and leaflets.

National Association For The Childless (NACK), 318 Summer Lane, Birmingham B19 3RL (021-359 4887).
Newsletter and regional groups.

National Childbirth Trust, 9 Queensborough Terrace, Bayswater, London W2 3TB.
Send SAE for information about work of NCT, about local groups (ante-natal preparation, post-natal support and breast-feeding counselling) and for list of publications and maternity sales.

National Council For One Parent Families, 255 Kentish Town Rd., London NW5 2LX (01-267 1361).
Advice and information. (A recent booklet, *Single and Pregnant*, gives details of the rights and maternity benefits for single parents.)

Pre-Eclamptic Toxaemia Society (PETS), Dawn James, 88 Plumberow, Lee Chapel North, Basildon, Essex SS15 5LP.
Regular newsletter, information and library service.

Pregnancy Sickness – for telephone counselling, 0943 609209 or 0851 5016.

Relaxation For Living, Dunesk, 29 Burwood Park Rd., Walton-on-Thames, Surrey, KT12 5LH. (09322 27826).
Information and reading list.

The Soil Association, Walnut Tree Manor, Haughley, Stowmarket, Suffolk (044 970235).
Information about local groups. Promotes fuller understanding of relationship between soil, plants, animals and man.

The Spastics Society, Publications and Information Department, 12 Park Crescent, London W1N 4EQ (01-636-5020).

Eating Well for a Healthy Pregnancy

Issues a series of consumer publications about health of parents and babies. (e.g. 'Healthy mother, healthy baby'). Free.

The Stillbirth And Neonatal Death Society (SANDS), Argyle House, 29–31 Euston Rd., London NW1 2SD. tel: 01-833 2851/2.
A network of local groups. Also has leaflets for bereaved parents.

Templegarth Trust, 82 Tinkle St., Grimoldby, Louth, Lincs LN11 8TF.
Produces leaflets (e.g. 'Starting Life Well', 70p + SAE).

The Twins Clubs Association, 'Porthladd', 27 Woodham Park Rd., Woodham, Weybridge, Surrey, KT15 3ST.
Gives support and encouragement to parents of twins; also produces leaflets for parents and a register of twins clubs.

The Vegan Society, 9 Mawddwy Cottages, Minllyn, Dinas Mawddwy, Machynlleth SY20 9LW. (06504 255).
For further information on vegan diets and experiences of vegan mothers.

The Vegetarian Society (UK) Ltd, 53 Marloes Rd., Kensington, London W8 6LA (01-937 7739).
For requests for further information.

Wholefood, 24 Paddington St., London W1M 4DR.
Bookshop; will send list of books available by post (on general nutrition and pregnancy and other aspects of health).

Women's Health Information Centre (WHIC), Ufton Centre, Ufton Rd., London N1 5BY.
Newsletter and information leaflets on wide range of issues relating to women's health.

Index

Alcohol 6, 9, 11, 79-81
Allergy 101, 119
Amenorrhoea 5, 39, 72, 73
Amniocentesis 97
Anaemia 105
Anencephaly 127
Animal studies 5, 9, 127
Aversions 92

Baby
    development of 1
    death 5, 103
    feeding 121
    food 119
    colic 115
    food sense 123
    refusal to eat 122
Beans, *see* Pulses
Biotin 30, 54, 56, 137
Birth interval, *see* Spacing
Birth weight 6, 103
Blood 2, 105
Blood pressure, *see* Hypertension
Body stores 2, 4, 86, 131
Bran 94, 108, 110
Bread 20, 60, 62
Breakfast 67
Breast-feeding 112, 116
    and alcohol 81
    and drugs 77
    and weight 47
    disadvantages of 113
Breast milk 112, 115
Butter 24

Caffeine 78
Calcium 2, 115, 134, 138
Calories 27, 100, 116
Carbohydrate 2, 33, 87
Carotene 22, 56, 136
Cereals 20, 60, 62, 120

Cheese 24, 61, 67, 120
Chemicals 10, 82
Chromium 139
Clinical assessment 130, 132
Codliver oil 74, 140
Coeliac disease 9
Coffee 35, 71, 78
Cola 78
Colostrum 114
Complementary proteins 98
Conception 5
Constipation 2, 94, 110
Contraception 73
Copper 138
Cottage cheese 24, 67
Cramps 95
Cravings 92
Cream 24
Cytomegalovirus 75

Deficiency 4, 125, 133
Diabetes 9, 42, 102
Diet 6
    daily 28
    low cost 55
Dietary analysis 130
Dietitian 27, 41, 101, 130
Diseases 9, 74
Diuretics 107
Down's syndrome 97
Drinks 35, 89, 117
Drugs 6, 10, 76

Eating patterns 67
Eating out 68
Economizing 55
Eggs 18, 59, 61
Embryo 2
Endocrine system 2
Enzymes 2

Index

Evidence 5, 125–8
Exercise 71
Experiments, see Research studies

Famine 5
Farming methods 15
Fat 2, 33, 100, 116
Fertility 5, 38, 71, 73
Fish 18, 59, 61, 75
Folate 2, 22, 30, 54, 105, 134, 137
Food
    additives 15, 55, 83
    cost of 51, 55
    fresh 14, 16
    groups of 16, 98, 112
    intolerance to 101
    labels 51, 83
    preparation 14, 16, 61
    sense 123
    storage 58
Formula milk 112
Freezer 50, 108, 121
Fruit 21, 60, 65, 120
    canned 23, 65
    dried 23, 65
    salad 65

Game 18
Genetics 1, 103
Genito-urinary diseases 75
German measles 75
Guidelines 13, 16, 25, 111

Haemoglobin 2, 78, 105
Handicap 5, 76, 103, 127
Healthy eating 13, 124
Heartburn 2, 94
Herbs 36
Herpes 75
Hormones 2, 86
Hospital 12, 108
Hyperemesis 85, 87
Hypertension 10, 42, 106

Ice-cream 66
Impotence 9, 71, 74
Industrial hazards 82
Infant foods 119
Infections 74, 113

Infertility 5, 8–10, 38, 73, 102, 105
Intra-uterine device (IUD) 74
Iron 2, 23, 30, 74, 100, 105, 114, 129, 134, 138

Juices, fruit and vegetable 23, 35, 90

Kelp 141

Labelling 51, 83
Laboratory tests 99, 105, 130, 132
Labour 109
Laxatives 94, 110
Lead 81–3
Leg cramps 95
Lentils, see Pulses
Let-down reflex 117
Liver 18, 61, 75, 83, 106, 141
Low-income 55

Magnesium 138
Male fertility 7–8
Malnutrition 4, 133
Manganese 139
Margarine 24
Meals 11, 28, 56, 67, 89
Meals out 68
Meat 17, 59, 61, 120
Medical disorders 9, 74, 103
Medicines 77
Mega-doses 74, 129
Men 7–12
Menstrual periods 5, 38–9, 71, 74
Milk 23, 61, 101, 120
Milk (human), see Breast milk
Milk let-down 117
Minerals 2, 6, 30–1, 35, 56, 74, 83, 100, 125, 138
Miscarriage 103, 105
Money 51, 55
Muesli, see Cereals
Mumps 9

Nausea 3, 6, 84
Niacin 30, 54, 56, 137
Nourishment 70
Nutritional status 130

Index

Nuts 19, 59, 99

Oedema 106
Older mothers 96
Organic food 15
Overconsumption 128
Ovum 1, 8

Pantothenic acid 30, 54, 56, 137
Pasta 21, 60, 63
Pastry 63
Peas, *see* Pulses
Pica 93
Pill 73
Placenta 3
Pollution 6, 81
Porridge, *see* Cereals
Portions 25, 27
Postnatal depression 111
Potatoes 60, 64
Poultry 18, 59
Preconception 5
Pre-eclampsia 106
Processed foods 15
Protein 2, 27, 87, 98
Ptyalism 93
Pulses 19, 59, 62, 99, 120

Quetelet index 8, 39

Radiation 82
Refined foods 14
Relaxation 6, 71, 72
   classes in 72, 108
Research studies 5, 9, 13, 123, 127
Rest 6, 72, 88, 117
Riboflavin 30, 54, 56, 61, 71, 73, 137
Rice 21, 60, 63

Salad 16, 22, 60, 63, 65
Saliva 93
Salt 35, 107, 121
Sea 15
Seeds 19, 99
Selenium 139
Shopping 11, 50, 51, 108
Sickness 2, 84
   mild 88
   severe 91
   and baby's sex 87
Single parent 55, 84
Slimming 37, 42
Smell 93
Smoking 6, 9, 11, 78
Soil 15
Soup 59, 64
Soy products 19, 99, 101
Spacing of pregnancies 6, 104
Sperm 1, 7
Spices 36, 68
Spina bifida 127
Sponge 109
Starvation 5, 38–9
Stillbirth 103
Stitches 110
Stock 14, 59
Storage of food 58
Stores, *see* Body stores
Stress 6, 42, 70, 87
Subfertility 102
Supplements 68, 125, 127–9, 141

Tea 35, 71, 78
Teenage pregnancy 96
Temperature 9
Testes 7–9
Thiamin 30, 54, 56, 137
Tiredness 72, 86
Toxoplasmosis 75
Twins 97

Undernutrition 5, 6, 133

Vegan diets 98
Vegetables 21, 60, 63, 120
Vegetarian diets 19, 98
Vitamins 2, 6, 30–1, 35, 54, 56, 73, 76, 83, 125, 135–7
   specific vitamins 30, 54, 56, 137
   charts of 30–1, 54, 56, 131, 135–7
   classification of 126
   vitamin B_6 2, 30, 54, 56, 73, 87, 92, 137
   vitamin B_{12} 30, 54, 56, 99, 137
   vitamin C 2, 22, 30, 54, 56, 65, 73, 74, 79, 100, 129, 137

Index

Vomiting 3, 85, 91

Weaning 118
Well-balanced diet 25
Weight 37, 85, 97
    after the birth 47
    before pregnancy 37
    chart 40
    desirable 39, 41
    gain in pregnancy 44
    losing weight 42, 85
    overweight 8, 41, 42, 46, 48
    underweight 39, 46, 48
Weights of food 32, 52, 55
Wheatgerm 60, 75, 140
Whole foods 14, 16
Work hazards 10, 82-3

X-rays 82

Yeast extracts 32, 55, 90, 141
Yogurt 24, 57, 66, 82, 120

Zinc 129, 138